Elizabeth Bowen and the Writing of Trauma

COSTERUS NEW SERIES 202

Series Editors:
C.C. Barfoot, László Sándor Chardonnens
and Theo D'haen

Elizabeth Bowen and the Writing of Trauma

The Ethics of Survival

Jessica Gildersleeve

Rodopi Amsterdam-New York, NY 2014

Cover image: Holland House library after an air raid in 1940. Reproduced by kind permission of English Heritage, BB83/04456 Library at Holland House.

Cover design: Aart Jan Bergshoeff

The paper on which this book is printed meets the requirements of "ISO 9706:1994, Information and documentation - Paper for documents - Requirements for permanence".

ISBN: 978-90-420-3799-1
E-Book ISBN: 978-94-012-1047-8

Printed in the Netherlands

Contents

ACKNOWLEDGEMENTS

I would like to thank the Harry Ransom Humanities Research Centre for permission to quote from works held in these archives. The cover image (depicting Holland House library after an air raid in 1940) is reproduced by kind permission of English Heritage.

Development of the following work was made possible at various stages by funding from the Overseas Research Students Award Scheme, a University of Bristol Postgraduate Research Scholarship, and the Faculty of Arts, University of Southern Queensland.

I am grateful to my colleagues at the University of Bristol, the University of Queensland, Griffith University, and the University of Southern Queensland, for the friendship, advice and intellectual support they have provided at different points during this project. In particular, I am indebted to Andrew Bennett, Jude Seaboyer, Ika Willis, Belinda McKay, Lesa Scholl, and Kezia Whiting. Finally, to Adam Kelly, and to Chris and Sue Gildersleeve – thank you.

INTRODUCTION

"WE MUST LIVE HOW WE CAN"

> I cannot really have felt you were dead, I think, because one doesn't go on talking and talking to any one of *them*: more one goes on hearing what they said, piecing and repiecing it together to try and make out something they had not time to say – possibly even had not had time to know. There still must be something that matters that one has forgotten, forgotten because at the time one did not realize how much it did matter. Yet most of all there is something one has got to forget – that is, if it is to be possible to live. The more wars there are, I suppose, the more we shall learn how to be survivors.[1]

> To live, by definition, is not something one learns. Not from oneself, it is not learned from life, taught by life. Only from the other and by death. In any case from the other at the edge of life.
>
> … The time of the "learning to live," a time without tutelary present, would amount to this, to which the exordium is leading us: to learn to live with ghosts, in the upkeep, the conversation, the company, or the companionship, in the commerce without commerce of ghosts.[2]

Trauma and survival

Writing trauma is always already constituted by survival: learning to live, learning how to survive. This is true for two main reasons. First, writing the traumatic event must testify to the author's survival, so that what has been seen and known is recorded. I live, the trauma survivor implies, to write; I write because I live. Second, writing

[1] Elizabeth Bowen, *The Heat of the Day* (1949), New York: Anchor, 2002, 358 (original emphasis). Hereafter cited parenthetically as *HD*.

[2] Jacques Derrida, *Spectres of Marx: The State of the Debt, the Work of Mourning, and the New International*, trans. Peggy Kamuf, New York: Routledge, 1994, xviii.

constitutes a form of survival: a form of bearing witness, of immortalization. The traumatic experience remains as a persistent presence, beyond forgetting, when it is in text. But writing trauma, so often described as "unspeakable", is never so simple. How should such events be recorded? Who may record them? Whose responsibility is it to record them? Survival, as Cathy Caruth suggests, is itself a crisis.[3]

In this book, I explore the work of Anglo-Irish author Elizabeth Bowen as a lifelong project of ethical representation and of understanding the narrative responsibilities of the survivor, and suggest that her work is most importantly seen as an example of the inextricability of twentieth-century literature, suffering, and bearing witness: "*We have to learn to survive*," Bowen asserts, "*while we learn to write*".[4] This is the crisis of survival, and a problem grappled with in each of Bowen's texts. This book attempts to do justice to the strangeness of Bowen's writing, and to Bowen's assertion that, "In a sense, it is fiction's business to *be* strange", in its concern with the ways in which writing survives, integrates (or fails to integrate), and represents trauma.[5] I argue that Bowen's writing is always and everywhere the narrative of trauma, and show that throughout her life she experimented with the methodology of trauma writing. More than this, I argue that her work is best understood through the lens of contemporary literary theory by Jacques Derrida, Hélène Cixous and Julia Kristeva because Bowen appears to anticipate their deconstructive projects. This means that alongside presenting close analyses of Bowen's fiction as trauma writing, this book implicitly traces an evolution of deconstructive thought throughout the twentieth century, and shows that this theoretical model is concomitant with an understanding of trauma narratives.

The field of trauma studies has been subject to an explosion of interest, in particular since the American Psychiatric Association's (APA) decision in 1980 to include Post-Traumatic Stress Disorder

---

[3] Cathy Caruth, "Introduction", in *Trauma: Explorations in Memory*, ed. Cathy Caruth, Baltimore, MD: Johns Hopkins University Press, 1995, 9.

[4] Elizabeth Bowen, "Sources of Influence" (1962), in *Elizabeth Bowen: A Study of the Short Fiction*, ed. Phyllis Lassner, New York: Twayne, 1991, 147 (original emphasis).

[5] Elizabeth Bowen, "Outrageous Ladies" (1949-63), in *People, Places, Things: Essays by Elizabeth Bowen*, ed. Allan Hepburn, Edinburgh: Edinburgh University Press, 2008, 379 (original emphasis).

(PTSD) in the Diagnostic and Statistical Manual of Mental Disorders (DSM-III-R). The discipline has been primarily influenced by Sigmund Freud's work, especially in *Beyond the Pleasure Principle* (1920) and *Mourning and Melancholia* (1917), where he explored this tendency of trauma survivors to suffer from recurring nightmares and the inexplicable repetition of previous events. More recently, Nicolas Abraham and Maria Torok's radical rereadings of Freud in *The Shell and the Kernel* (1972) and *The Wolf Man's Magic Word* (1976) have extended the importance of this paradigm for literary studies. These psychoanalytic models propose that trauma is a kind of psychological wounding caused by an event so extreme that it cannot be immediately assimilated, and is thus, paradoxically, only first experienced in its repetition, and as a function of its forgetting. Freud explained the uncontrollable recurrences of the traumatic event as the "repetition compulsion", and argued that the trauma survivor is compelled to re-enact the event until it has been "worked through" – until the strangely "forgotten" event has been recognized and integrated into the survivor's life narrative. This means, then, that trauma is not limited to the originating event, but rather is more clearly characterized by its spectral return, "in the way that its very unassimilated nature – the way it was precisely *not known* in the first instance – returns to haunt the survivor later on".[6]

Contemporary trauma studies (particularly in the context of Holocaust studies, which dominate the field) seek to elucidate the ways in which, as Roger Luckhurst has noted, "psychoanalysis and literature are particularly privileged forms of writing" that are able to attend to trauma's "perplexing paradoxes".[7] Indeed, it seems as if the study of memory has been subsumed by the study of trauma, as increasingly, recognize Paul Antze and Michael Lambek, "memory worth talking about – worth remembering – is memory of trauma".[8] In this context, Caruth has emerged as the most powerful critical voice in contemporary trauma studies; her work in *Trauma: Explorations in*

---

[6] Cathy Caruth, *Unclaimed Experience: Trauma, Narrative, and History*, Baltimore, MD: Johns Hopkins University Press, 1996, 4 (original emphasis).

[7] Roger Luckhurst, *The Trauma Question*, London: Routledge, 2008, 5.

[8] Paul Antze and Michael Lambek, "Forecasting Memory", in *Tense Past: Cultural Essays in Trauma and Memory*, eds Paul Antze and Michael Lambek, New York: Routledge, 1996, xii.

Memory (1995) and, in particular, in *Unclaimed Experience: Trauma, Narrative, and History* (1996) (a work heavily indebted to Freud), remains the shaping force for studies of trauma in literary criticism. For Caruth, it is the very belatedness of its experience which characterizes the traumatic event. As she recognizes: "The historical power of the trauma is not just that the experience is repeated after its forgetting, but that it is only in and through its inherent forgetting that it is first experienced at all."[9]

It is in this sense of trauma as exceeding experience, as an event which one "had not had time to know", to recall my epigraph from Bowen's *The Heat of the Day* (1949), that Caruth's thinking about trauma is most important for the present study and for an analysis of Bowen's fiction, precisely because Caruth's understanding of trauma has affinities with Bowen's. Indeed, a skill by which Bowen "remained impressed", she once stated, was "people's formidable capacity for silence, for keeping a secret, and not less by their power of acting up, of behaving as though nothing were the matter".[10] This is evident, for example, in a draft of her 1952 Preface to *The Last September* (1929):

> I had in my early youth, experience ~~which had been less than half~~ little or less than conscious, little or never registered ~~by or analysed~~ by the mind, ~~at the time of happening~~, and therefore ~~till now remaining, in an indifferent "somewhere" of my memory, wonderfully unspoiled~~ immune and pure.
>
> … [The one who remembers] ~~can but be magnetised~~ back to those scenes ~~and times~~ of his own life most steeped in subjective experience which he did not know of. Sensation accumulates ~~where it is least sought, meaning flows in where we had imagined none, one is drawn by the mysterious hauntedness of a period not understood in its own time~~, retrospectively, where we were blind to any. One is captured by the mysterious the imperious hauntedness of a period not understood in its own time.[11]

---

[9] Caruth, "Introduction", 8.

[10] Elizabeth Bowen, "Elizabeth Bowen and Jocelyn Brooke in Conversation" (broadcast 3 October 1950), Harry Ransom Humanities Research Centre, Elizabeth Bowen Collection (HRHRC), 2.3, 13.

[11] Elizabeth Bowen, draft of Preface to *The Last September* (n.d.), HRHRC, 7.2, 2, 5. This text is struck through as in the original.

Bowen's fiction is conditioned by this "hauntedness" of the traumatic experience, an event "not understood in its own time" but stored in memory's "indifferent 'somewhere'". Her work is circumscribed by this sense of "belatedness", "hauntedness", "afterwardsness" or, more precisely, "deferred action" – what Freud terms *Nachträglichkeit*.[12] Time, in Bowen, is never "so simple as all that" (*HD* 283, 285, 303), and in this book I explore those temporal disruptions and disjunctions in Bowen's writing as characteristic of traumatic memory.

Trauma theory has not only influenced memory studies. As Eric L. Santner states, the language of trauma studies has similarly infiltrated "the semantic field" of critical theory in terms of what he calls a "rhetoric of mourning" – that is, "the recurrence, in so many postmodern theoretical discourses, of a metaphorics of loss and impoverishment", and of an appeal in those discourses "to notions of shattering, rupture, mutilation, fragmentation, to images of fissures, wounds, rifts, gaps, and abysses" – terms which have become synonymous with trauma.[13] This rhetoric describes much of the work of Derrida, Cixous and Kristeva. It is for this reason that their theoretical discourses are both anticipated by and find such resonance in Bowen's fiction. Throughout this book I draw on writing by these theorists not only in order to elucidate my thinking about Bowen's work as the writing of trauma, but to draw her prose into the lexical framework of this "rhetoric of mourning". Rather than simply applying such theory to Bowen's text, this book suggests that reading Bowen's fiction alongside deconstructive theory enables further understanding of the intersections between trauma and narrative that seek to extend a Freudian elucidation of mourning; the emergence of Bowen's methodology of trauma writing attends not only to an ethics of representation, but to the "hauntedness", or the traumatization, of language itself.

This book therefore seeks to move beyond what Anne Whitehead describes as the typical "paradox or contradiction" of trauma narratives – that is, "if trauma comprises an event or experience which

---

[12] Noting that Freud never entirely elucidated this concept, Nicola King provides a useful overview of *Nachträglichkeit* in her work: *Memory, Narrative, Identity: Remembering the Self*, Edinburgh: Edinburgh University Press, 2000, 4, 11.

[13] Eric L. Santner, *Stranded Objects: Mourning, Memory, and Film in Postwar Germany*, Ithaca, NY: Cornell University Press, 1990, 7.

overwhelms the individual and resists language or representation, how then can it be narrativized in fiction?"[14] It demonstrates the insufficiency of Dominick LaCapra's argument that "there is no such thing as writing trauma itself if only because trauma, while at times related to particular events, cannot be localized in terms of a discrete, dated experience".[15] Instead, it is concerned with the ways in which Bowen's writing survives trauma and works towards its ethical representation. In Bowen's writing we find language "asserted as that which can realize trauma even as it is theorized as that which fails in the face of trauma".[16]

Bowen's traumas

Bowen's writing is particularly sensitive to personal and cultural trauma partly because her own life was so clearly scarred by recurring traumatic events. She was born Elizabeth Dorothea Cole Bowen, at 15 Herbert Place in Dublin in 1899. She was an only child, and until the winter of her seventh year, she and her parents, Florence and Henry Cole Bowen, divided their time between this city residence and the family's ancestral home, Bowen's Court, in County Cork. Her memoir, *Seven Winters* (1942), records this time as "the essence of a beginning", for at seven years old Bowen experienced the first of those traumatic events which marked her life and which are compulsively repeated in her writing.[17] Henry Bowen was a barrister, and under some professional and financial stress. In the summer of 1905, he began to suffer from a mental illness diagnosed at the time as "anaemia of the brain". Over the next year, despite treatment, he grew worse, even becoming violent. Florence was unable to cope with his erratic behaviour, and with the pressure of managing the family's affairs alone, and so she was advised to leave Ireland. In the winter of 1906, she and "Bitha" (as the young Elizabeth was known) travelled to Kent, in England, to live with Florence's cousins while Henry recovered. They stayed in Kent until Bowen was thirteen, and

[14] Anne Whitehead, *Trauma Fiction*, Edinburgh: Edinburgh University Press, 2004, 3.
[15] Dominick LaCapra, *Writing History, Writing Trauma*, Baltimore, MD: Johns Hopkins University Press, 2001, 186.
[16] Leigh Gilmore, *The Limits of Autobiography: Trauma and Testimony*, Ithaca, NY: Cornell University Press, 2001, 7.
[17] Elizabeth Bowen, *Seven Winters* (1942), London: Longmans, 1943, 48.

After the war, the increased financial strain involved with the upkeep of Bowen's Court meant that Bowen began to take on more commissioned work for magazines, as well as lecture tours of America. In 1952 her husband died, and although she attempted to stay on at Bowen's Court, seeing it, now, as her only home, by 1959, overwhelmed by the cost and responsibility, she had decided to sell it. She accepted an offer from a local farmer, choosing to believe that the house would once again be filled with children; its new owner, however, had purchased the property for the land, and the house, which had so resolutely survived the Irish Troubles, was unceremoniously demolished. Bowen moved to the south of England, where she had once been so happy with her mother. Her last three novels, dealt with in the final chapters of this book, are all concerned with memory and memorialization: haunted by the place to which she had compulsively returned, in *A World of Love* (1958), *The Little Girls* (1963) and *Eva Trout, or Changing Scenes* (1968), Bowen tries to explore and to narrate the processes of traumatic memory, and the continuing influence of the past on the present. She continued to travel, lecture, and write until her death of lung cancer in 1973.

"We must live how we can"

The fact that her own life was irrevocably punctuated by personal and cultural traumatic events may be one reason why Bowen's work is so concerned with trauma, but also why a remarkable (and hitherto overlooked) recurrence in Bowen's fiction and non-fiction is an imperative to "live how one can"; to live, perhaps, around trauma, around that unknowable, unnameable "something" which "one has got to forget – that is, if it is to be possible to live". In *Friends and Relations*, Bowen's third novel (and a text far too often neglected by critics), this is emphasized by Janet when she insists that "we must all live *somehow*", and the sentiment is later echoed by her husband Rodney: "life has really got to be lived somehow."[23] In Bowen's next novel, *To the North*, Cecilia, "a little dwarfed" by the death of her husband, is emotionally amnesiac, unable to "estimate now what she suffered then: the sombre memory went beyond her compass". After trauma, Cecilia is sensationally impoverished, subject to "meaner

[23] Elizabeth Bowen, *Friends and Relations* (1931), Harmondsworth: Penguin, 1943, 24, 65. Hereafter cited parenthetically as *FR*.

living". In this novel, that "somehow" of *Friends and Relations* has been qualified; now, "*one has to live how one can*".[24]

This sense of being reduced or "dwarfed" by trauma reappears a few years later in Bowen's 1936 Preface to *The Faber Book of Modern Short Stories*, in which she suggests that it is fiction which might provide a "compensation" for this kind of "meaner living":

> The retreat from fact that private fantasy offers has been as grateful in life as its variations are fascinating to art. *Man has to live how he can*: overlooked and dwarfed he makes himself his own theatre.[25]

The Death of the Heart may be seen to follow on from *To the North* in the sense that Cecilia's "frightened heart" which "repairs itself in small ways" after the loss of her lover becomes the title trauma of the later novel (*TN* 99). *The Death of the Heart* repeats the strange phrase in its imperative to "defend ourselves against that terrible memory that is stronger than will .... We desert those who desert us; we cannot afford to suffer; *we must live how we can*".[26] The cost of suffering thus again implies meaner living, as it also does in another of Bowen's essays, in which she writes, in response to the claim that "One must live in the moment; one must seize what one can!": "What one can – how much that is precious eludes the too-hurried grasp!"[27]

In the post-war essay "Ireland", living "how one can" becomes part of the condition of living in a nation of civil unrest: "In whatever country, *one must live how one can*: it may be seen why Ireland lives as she does."[28] And when the imperative appears again, in *The Heat of the Day*, this kind of meagre survival can mean failing to live up to the expectations of, or to learn to live with, the dead:

---

[24] Elizabeth Bowen, *To the North* (1932), London: Vintage, 1999, 99 (emphasis added). Hereafter cited parenthetically as *TN*.

[25] Elizabeth Bowen, "Preface to *The Faber Book of Modern Short Stories*" (1936), in *Collected Impressions*, London: Longmans Green, 1950, 44 (emphasis added). This sense of fantasy as a "compensation" or "retreat" is particularly evident, I argue in Chapter Five, in Bowen's wartime short fiction.

[26] Elizabeth Bowen, *The Death of the Heart* (1938), New York: Anchor, 2000, 190-91 (emphasis added). Hereafter cited parenthetically as *DH*. This kind of psychological defence in *The Death of the Heart* is the focus of Chapter Four.

[27] Elizabeth Bowen, "The Art of Respecting Boundaries" (1952), in *People, Places, Things*, 399.

[28] Elizabeth Bowen, "Ireland" (n.d.), HRHRC, 6.5, 20 (emphasis added).

> One must not be too much influenced by a dead person! After all, *one can only live how one can*; one generally finds there is only one way one *can* live – and that often must mean disappointing the dead. They had no idea how it would be for us. If they still had to live, who knows that they might not have disappointed themselves? (*HD* 96; emphasis added)

From *The Heat of the Day* on, disappointment taints this iterated obligation, and it ultimately mutates, in Bowen's final novel, *Eva Trout, or Changing Scenes*, into explosive resentment towards the responsibilities that survival entails:

> "I wonder," [Henry] said, "whether, in spite of all I was telling you this morning, you *can* conceive what a state I am in and how chaotic it is. *Feel*? – I refuse to; that would be the last straw! There's too much of everything, yet nothing. Is it the world, or what? Everything's hanging over one. The expectations one's bound to disappoint. The dread of misfiring. The knowing there's something one can't stave off. The Bomb is the least. Look what's got to happen to us if we do live, look at the results! Living is brutalizing: just look at everybody! We shan't simply toughen, Eva, we shall grossen."[29]

In *Eva Trout*, survival may no longer be worth the cost, if the "results" of living "how one can" mean that one is not living, but rather, in Bowen's strange verbal alignment, "brutalizing". Throughout this book, I consider how such refusal of feeling moves beyond "toughen[ing]" to a "grossen[ing]" not just of life, but of narrative language itself: a deepening, enlarging, or monstrification of language that I read as the writing of trauma.

[29] Elizabeth Bowen, *Eva Trout, or Changing Scenes* (1968), New York: Anchor, 2003, 262 (original emphasis). Hereafter cited parenthetically as *ET*.

CHAPTER 1

WOUND: *THE HOTEL* AND *TO THE NORTH*

> Once the wound closes up we speak of it no longer, but we never forget it.[1]

> Across the mind's surface – on which a world's apprehension, strain at home and in Europe, were gravely written – the sense of a spoilt summer, so much prettiness wasted, darkly spread like spilt ink. (*TN* 177)

The term "trauma" is derived from the Greek *τραῦμα*, a "wound".[2] When we speak of those suffering from trauma, or of a textual representation of trauma, we speak of a psychological wound, the scar or mark of a painful event. "Traumatisms", or stigmata, pierce character, time, and text so that, as Caruth points out, this "wound of the mind" figures a "breach in the mind's experience of time, self, and the world".[3] Caruth introduces her work on cultural trauma theory in reference to Freud's *Beyond the Pleasure Principle*, and his reading of Tasso's *Gerusalemme Liberata*, in which a soldier unwittingly kills his lover, and later wounds her again when he hears her soul, imprisoned in a tree, cry out. For Caruth, Tasso's tale "evocatively represent[s] in Freud's text the way that the experience of a trauma repeats itself, exactly and unremittingly, through the unknowing acts of the survivor and against his very will".[4] It is only in its repetition, Caruth and Freud both point out, that the traumatic event can be known; the wound, then, is at once the traumatic act which was hidden from conscious thought, and the very means by which it is recalled.

---

[1] Hélène Cixous, "What Is It O'Clock? Or the Door (We Never Enter)" (1994), trans. Catherine A.F. MacGillivray, in *Stigmata: Escaping Texts*, London: Routledge, 2005, 84.

[2] See "trauma", *OED Online* (accessed 11 November 2009).

[3] Jacques Derrida, "Foreword", trans. Eric Prenowitz, in Cixous, *Stigmata*, ix-x.

[4] Caruth, *Unclaimed Experience*, 2.

Both *The Hotel* and *To the North* are concerned with this “wound” or “breach” of “time, self, and the world”. The climax of each novel involves a car crash (one wished for, the other actually occurring). While in the former text Sydney approaches the abyss of traumatic recognition before stopping short at its edge, in the latter novel Emmeline propels herself to destruction. Criticism of *To the North* has often addressed this novel as tragedy.[5] What I want to suggest is that Emmeline’s final act of self-destruction, and Sydney’s desire for the same, is a function of trauma: Emmeline and Sydney are characterized by, and act in response to and as a result of, their psychological wounds. What we are asked to pay attention to in these novels is not only the physical abyss which yawns before these characters, but that which is present inside them, the voice which cries out from the wound. It is in such “crying-out theme[s] of suffering-horror”, as Kristeva terms them, that narrative and narrated identity collapse.[6] The emptiness which characterizes the descriptions of both Emmeline and Sydney as they hover on the brink of destruction figures the abjection which characterizes “suffering-horror”, that is, the traumatic recognition of the weeping, wounded self.

Traumatic suspension

To the North juxtaposes Cecilia and Emmeline Summers, sisters-in-law bound by the late Henry, Cecilia’s husband and Emmeline’s brother. The pair are reminiscent of the Pinkertons of *The Hotel*, Bowen’s first novel, a widow and a bereaved sister with whom the lost husband and brother perpetually “mak[es] a third”: “this evening as ever, his mild be-whiskered face, with that expression of awe on it with which fancy is wont to invest the pictured faces of the dead, looked out from a vast scrolled frame that overshadowed the silver-stoppered bottles on the dressing-table.”[7] In *To the North*, however,

---

[5] See, for example, Andrew Bennett and Nicholas Royle, *Elizabeth Bowen and the Dissolution of the Novel*, London: Macmillan, 1995, 24; John Coates, *Social Discontinuity in the Novels of Elizabeth Bowen: The Conservative Quest*, New York: Edwin Mellen, 1998, 77, 97; Hermione Lee, *Elizabeth Bowen*, rev. edn, London: Vintage, 1999, 71.

[6] Julia Kristeva, *Powers of Horror: An Essay on Abjection*, trans. Leon S. Roudiez, New York: Columbia University Press, 1982, 141.

[7] Elizabeth Bowen, *The Hotel* (1927), London: Penguin, 1987, 24. Hereafter cited parenthetically as *TH*. See also Maud Ellmann, *The Shadow Across the Page*,

the lost third is not so obviously present: rather than being immortalized and adored, the dead Henry is only a site of pain and absence.

Since Henry's death, Cecilia and Emmeline have set up a house together on Oudenarde Road, in St John's Wood. The women cohabit in spite of the disapproval of their shared relation, Lady Waters, who is certain that:

> Women could not live together, sisters-in-law especially. How much did they speak of Henry, how lively a bond was their loss? (*Ibid.*, 13)

Bowen is uncharacteristically specific regarding the detail of Cecilia and Emmeline's address; perhaps symbolic of their relationship, as well as of each woman's traumatic repression, the site suggests an impression of luxury and control masking embattled depths. As such, the novel opens on the happiness and convenience of the women's shared home, a refuge for them both – for Cecilia, from a whirl of social engagements and travel, and for Emmeline, who runs a travel agency, a space distant from the demands of managing her business, its difficult clients, and her even more difficult colleagues. By chance, Cecilia meets Mark Linkwater on a train from Milan to London; the romantic relationship which develops between Markie and Emmeline sets in motion the tragic arc of the narrative. The heterosexual romances of both women disrupt their domestic idyll, for Cecilia's eventual decision to marry Julian Tower awakens in Emmeline the recognition that "Houses shared with women are built on sand" (*ibid.*, 208). Indeed, it appears that the lives and livelihoods of the two women have, as Lady Waters suspected, been built on loss, shown to be a precarious foundation that must ultimately give way. Emmeline's discovery of Markie's infidelity shortly after the news of Cecilia's engagement destroys the calm established at the novel's introduction. In its closing scenes, the wounds of the narrative gape: Emmeline drives herself and Markie headlong into annihilation, while Cecilia and Julian are left in suspense, waiting for Emmeline's impossible return.

Edinburgh: Edinburgh University Press, 99; Heather Bryant Jordan, *How Will the Heart Endure: Elizabeth Bowen and the Landscape of War*, Ann Arbor: University of Michigan Press, 1992, 27.

To the North overlays the political with the personal. To return to this chapter's epigraph, the "world's apprehension" of "strain" (including the possibility of another war) is "gravely written" across the collective mind, while Emmeline Summers might herself be understood to be the "spoilt summer", the "wasted" "prettiness" which spreads "like spilt ink". Vera Kreilkamp notes that although wartime "losses" are, in this novel, "virtually unmentioned", they "shadow a post-war edginess".[8] In *To the North*, she argues, "the First World War exists not only as a dislocating break with the past, but as the century's recurring source of the dead, the maimed and ghostly undead".[9] Later, Bowen's writing during the Second World War makes clear that recurrence – this is a wounding doomed, like Tasso's wounding of Clorinda, to be repeated. In the 1941 short story, "Tears, Idle Tears", for example, the eyes of the child, Frederick, and of the adult, George, are figured as "wounds, in the world's surface, through which its inner, terrible unassuageable, necessary sorrow constantly bled away and as constantly welled up".[10] Almost like a tide, the story suggests, blood and tears will be spilled, over and over. In this chapter, I argue that what I see as Emmeline's death-in-livingness is symptomatic of the aftermath of war: she represents the wounding, or the woundedness, of her generation, as one of "the maimed and ghostly undead".

To the North is a text which bears "the trace of a wound".[11] While the novel does not explicitly engage with the events or effects of the First World War (the only overt reference documents the reaction of Cecilia's mother to the deaths of her soldier sons [*ibid.*, 13]), it nevertheless "translate[s]" the physical and psychological wounds of war into the text itself. *To the North* is almost scarred by the unacknowledged war; it bears the trace or mark of a particular place and time: the First World War. As Heather Bryant Jordan has recognized, in spite of its "sustained influence" upon Bowen's life, the

---

[8] Vera Kreilkamp, "Bowen: Ascendancy Modernist", in *Elizabeth Bowen*, ed. Eibhear Walshe, Dublin: Irish Academic Press, 2009, 19. See also Jordan, *How Will the Heart Endure*, 23; Bennett and Royle, *Elizabeth Bowen and the Dissolution of the Novel*, 35.

[9] Kreilkamp, "Bowen: Ascendancy Modernist", 19.

[10] Elizabeth Bowen, "Tears, Idle Tears" (1941), in *The Collected Stories of Elizabeth Bowen*, ed. Angus Wilson, London: Vintage, 1999, 486.

[11] Hélène Cixous, "Preface: On Stigmatexts", trans. Eric Prenowitz, in Cixous, *Stigmata*, xi.

First World War only ever enters her work "by way of shadows and hints and reproving glances from handsome young men in frames on mantelpieces", and "remains a steady but saddening fact that lonely women and injured men must acknowledge, whether they wish to or not".[12] But more than this kind of thematic absent presence, I suggest that this war (and later, World War Two) effects a textual wounding which can be traced throughout Bowen's work, and may be said to constitute her writing of trauma. In the sense that all of Bowen's work occurs in the aftermath of, or indeed during, war, to speak of textual trauma in *To the North* and elsewhere is to speak of the ways in which Bowen's writing is marked by the past and to consider the means by which her narratives bear or reinscribe the wounds of history and memory.

Henry Summers' death is the impetus for the novel's action.[13] As in *The Hotel*, from the shrine of his frame, in the heart of the house on Oudenarde Road, Henry forms the dead centre of *To the North*, the space of loss to which Cecilia and Emmeline react. Henry, stopped short, caught in a "fixed … half-look that in life was so rare and fleeting", can be read as a figure for stilled or suspended time in this novel. That is, his death comes to represent not only an emotional wounding of Cecilia and Emmeline, but a gash in the very temporality of the narrative, figuring a site of traumatic preservation. Indeed, it seems to be the suddenness of Henry's death, his sudden stillness, which unnerves and "disconcert[s]" (*ibid*., 29) Cecilia, who is like the "widowed shepherdess with only the clock to smile at" (*ibid*., 20): "bewildered", incredulous, she does "not know where to turn" (*ibid*., 13).

Cecilia's restlessness, her yearning for travel, her penchant for strangers and for strangeness, enacts a jittery desire to escape this centre of stillness.[14] But this is something more than the restlessness which Lady Waters identifies as a social affliction during this period between the two world wars:

---

[12] Jordan, *How Will the Heart Endure*, 18.

[13] It is Henry's death which provokes his widow and sister to move "to the north", to the house in St John's Wood, North London (Ellmann, *The Shadow Across the Page*, 99).

[14] Cecilia "loved strangers, strangeness …. Dim with her ignorance, lit by her fancy, any stranger went straight to her head" (*ibid*., 8).

> All ages are restless .... But *this* age ... is far more than restless: it is decentralized. From week to week, there is no knowing where anyone is. (*Ibid.*, 170)

For Cecilia, "decentralization" becomes a refusal of the literal dead centre, the staring photograph and the "coffer of ashes" which memorialize the stilling of her own plot (*ibid.*, 160). Cecilia's wish to live with her mother in America, for example, is born of this rejection of the past:

> No more summer ghosts, no belated cuckoo deforming all the remembered sweetness of spring in his spoilt cry. In that continent bare of her youth she saw herself as a girl again. He won't come with me, she thought of Henry; we shall forget one another, she thought of Julian .... Strangers, the kindly touch of the unforeseen – it was high time she was abroad again. The heart is a little thing and one can coerce it; she would step up the cheerful gangway and go abroad ... so one leaves behind one's little coffer of ashes. (*Ibid.*, 159-60)

Cecilia longs for more than a change of scene: what she wants is to return to a time prior to her marriage, to the shelter of her mother's household, to that spring of her girlhood before she became a Summers. Her escape from the "little coffer of ashes", and from the "morgue" of memories at Farraways (which gruesomely "lay with their faces upturned" [*ibid.*, 161]), is thus not only a means of distancing herself from this oppressive stillness, archive of death, but to precede it, to cheat the wounding of her expected narrative:

> Here she was at a standstill, her plot only half spun out .... It could not always be Henry.
>
> Emmeline knew it was not, still, Henry, but was his death. More shocked by this than she knew, a little dwarfed by the accident, Cecilia could not estimate now what she suffered then: the sombre memory went beyond her compass. Death gone, one rejects the ordeal instantly: grief, great in momentous passing, leaves one a little smaller. Obstinate in its refusal to suffer, the spirit puts up defences; the frightened heart repairs itself in small ways. Very few remain ennobled; one has to live how one can .... (*Ibid.*, 99)[15]

[15] This important passage is very often overlooked in favour of its succeeding metaphor of the "great house ... destroyed by fire" (*ibid.*, 99). Lee, for example,

It is "not, still, Henry", which thwarts Cecilia's "plot", but still Henry, dead Henry, in whom she can yet barely believe, the ghost with whom she lies, and who weighs her down even as she tries to flee. Cecilia's means of survival, then, is to attempt to spurn Henry's death by temporally circumventing its very occurrence, to "[reject] the ordeal" and "refus[e] to suffer".

This passage anticipates *The Death of the Heart*, and that novel's assertion that, "We desert those who desert us; we cannot afford to suffer; we must live how we can" (*DH* 191). Cecilia is a precursor to Anna Quayne, in the later novel; the assertion that "Disability seems a hard reward for courage" applies equally to both women, a stilled heart poor compensation for avoiding grief (*TN* 100). Later, Cecilia's "refusal to suffer" is reiterated, for her "alliance [with Emmeline] remained, on Cecilia's side certainly, largely defensive. Henry's death had been something ravaging, disproportionate; around Oudenarde Road a kind of pale was put up against one kind of emotion: nothing on that scale was to occur again" (*ibid.*, 148). However, rather than putting into practice the numbness of "death sleep", as Anna does, Cecilia adopts a frenzied restlessness which denies this dead stillness in her past, and makes certain that "nothing on that scale [will] occur again". Cecilia refuses to be stopped (by the) dead – a consequence which, from the novel's opening, it is made clear she dreads:

> At Chiasso, they stopped dead, it appeared forever .... As the wait prolonged itself and a kind of dull tension became apparent, she sent one wild comprehensive glance round her fellow travellers, as though less happy than cattle, conscious, they were all going to execution. (*Ibid.*, 5)

In the novel's final scene, however, cruelly and terribly, Cecilia, who so fears stillness, is condemned to forever await Emmeline in the hallway of their home, suspended in the threshold of the novel, and held on the threshold of advancing her own narrative, caught in the open wound of her sister-in-law's absence. For Cixous, these kinds of "flight[s] in the face of the intolerable" have a further effect, for in

---

suggests that such "landscapes of dereliction are made to illustrate states of mind" (*Elizabeth Bowen*, 76). See also Coates, *Social Discontinuity in the Novels of Elizabeth Bowen*, 73; Kreilkamp, "Bowen: Ascendancy Modernist", 15.

"fleeing", she argues, "the flight *saves* the trace of what it flees. This is why they flee: to *maintain* the horror *unforgettable* – the horror we would not live in the present although we want to keep its awful treasure, its proof, its testimony, its transfiguration."[16] In escaping, one must always refer back to "the trace" of what is fled, determining, saving and reinscribing this as a centre, an unforgettable but precious wound, even as it is left behind. Cecilia's frantic movement, then, may be read as a physical enactment of the processes of traumatic memory, at once seeking to save and to reject "the trace" of Henry's death, to preserve it in a stilled space outside of time, even as she works to escape its influence.

The photograph of Henry which "dominate[s]" Cecilia's mantelpiece makes this clear. It also, however, points up an important association of Henry with Emmeline (*ibid.*, 29):

> Sometimes – by those queer interchanges when [Cecilia] sat most alone, in the cold widowed solitude of her room – their whole married year seemed annulled; sometimes it seemed they had not been lovers ... Henry looked at you like Emmeline, but more guardedly, more satirically. You read the same skating quickness of thought, less resolution, more feeling, the same reluctance or inability to engage oneself closely with life on any terms. In spite of an almost fantastic detachment of manner and delicate frame, Henry had shown more vigour and less detachment than Emmeline – had he not married Cecilia? (*Ibid.*, 30)

The eerie slippage to second-person narration in this passage not only emphasizes the unity of the Summers siblings, who possess an affinity exacerbated by their orphanhood – "They brought themselves up side by side, Henry some years ahead; very much alike, as though the same tree had divided" – but an enforced concordance of the reader with Cecilia (*ibid.*, 13). Moreover, the instruction "You read" provides a temporal ambiguity (at once past and present tense) which simultaneously looks back to a time when one could read Henry, and conveys an immediacy which brings him back to life, thus functioning like the photograph itself. The final question mark underscores the "incredulity" which shadows Cecilia's marriage and widowhood; that

[16] Cixous, "On Stigmatexts", xi (original emphasis).

"married year" now seems impossible, "annulled" (*ibid.*, 13). Annulment constitutes erasure, present here in the ellipses which follow the question of the couple ever having been lovers; annulment represents a voiding of legal memory which enables a return to a state prior to the event. Annulment, therefore, comes to figure the unknownness of traumatic memory.

Emmeline, too, is fatally propelled by her brother's death. However, unlike Cecilia, who flees the stilled heart, Emmeline is rather pulled or magnetized into the vacuum of *To the North*'s dead centre. The affinity between Emmeline and her brother (reinforced throughout the narrative), in addition to her orphaned abandonment and subsequent sense of unbelonging, brings about in Emmeline a desire for a dissolution of the self which would unite her with her lost brother. Andrew Bennett and Nicholas Royle have argued that it is the "desire for death … which seems to be embodied by Emmeline, to embody her", and they trace this to "a desire for the stillness of death", an "aspiration towards the condition of still life".[17] However, I propose that it is precisely Emmeline's "stillness", constituted as a kind of detachment from life, which foreshadows the narrative climax of her death. The conclusion figures the culminating moment of the novel in which Emmeline's psychological detachment is aligned with her physical state. In this final act of self-harm, Emmeline unifies the destruction of her physical body with her psychological wounds.

Emmeline's stillness or detachment from life (shared by Henry), could also be read as a means of defence similar to Anna Quayne's "death sleep" which, in *The Death of the Heart*, provides protection from further wounding. Hers is a psychological condition typical of those in recoil from the First World War, and her rush for death is perhaps best understood as a fantasy of escape, "a healing stillness that had eluded her happy and living" (*ibid.*, 242), so that she is now "perplexed by the absence of pain" (*ibid.*, 244). On the one hand, suicide might become a way to insure herself against further hurt, after the pain caused by the callous Markie. However, it is not solely in response to Markie's infidelity that Emmeline drives them to their deaths – indeed, it is her sense of abandonment after Cecilia announces her engagement which incites in Emmeline the thought that she "and what was left of Henry must draw in closer" (*ibid.*, 213). Her

---

[17] Bennett and Royle, *Elizabeth Bowen and the Dissolution of the Novel*, 27, 28.

affair with Markie actually delays her desire for dissolution or "dematerializ[ation]" (*ibid.*, 67) and oneness with Henry; the rather modern psychic vacancy which Markie has throughout the novel recognized and feared in Emmeline is, in these final scenes, made sense of: "she turned his way, after a moment of silence, that same dilated and musing look of inquiry that, breaking again and again across their intimacy, had made him feel her no more than delayed on a journey elsewhere" (*ibid.*, 243). This, then, rather than the tragic or "fatal momentum of the narrative" would be the sense of predestination, the compulsion to repeat, the impression that "every door leads to death" (*ibid.*, 185), to which it is possible Bowen referred when she lamented: "Poor Emmeline! … It was inevitable."[18] Emmeline's death "wouldn't … be very noticeable" (*TN* 192) because, in a sense, it is "already as though she did not exist" – her psychic suspension works as a precursor to her physical absence (*ibid.*, 175). The novel's conclusion thus marks the only point at which Emmeline's physical state mirrors her psychological disintegration. Her death thus allows her alignment (or her reunion) with Henry, as well as the symmetry of her own psychic and physical conditions.

Emmeline's withdrawal from life is made clear throughout the novel; she is described as "transparent" (*ibid.*, 56, 137), "elsewhere" (*ibid.*, 122), "like a ghost astray" (*ibid.*, 66-67), "a stranger" (*ibid.*, 148). When Markie speaks to her, she psychologically retreats: "She had gone away" (*ibid.*, 194). Most striking, perhaps, is the insistence that she is an "angel" (*ibid.*, 243) or "inhuman" (*ibid.*, 120).[19] Critics often juxtapose these with equally frequent descriptions of Markie as "reptilian" or demonic, at times condemning Bowen for falling into a trap of metaphorical simplicity (*ibid.*, 7, 44).[20] However, I suggest that

[18] Bowen, cited in Glendinning, *Elizabeth Bowen: Portrait of a Writer*, 86.

[19] See, for example, Lee, who suggests that "there's some strain felt in the effort to load Emmeline and Markie's relationship with elemental imagery and ominous images of travel" (*Elizabeth Bowen*, 68-70). William Heath complains that Emmeline is given the title of "angel" with an "almost annoying frequency" ("The Jacobean Melodrama of *To the North*", in *Elizabeth Bowen*, ed. Harold Bloom, New York: Chelsea House, 1987, 29).

[20] See, for example, Heath (*ibid.*, 29). I have found no suggestion, however, that one might read Emmeline's "snake-skin shoes" as a signifier of her fall to the charms and influence of serpentine Markie (*TN* 53).

it is possible to read Emmeline's "angelicness" and inhumanity not, or not only, as representations of innocence or goodness, but as a Modernist anxiety about one's proximity to death, an "inability to engage … closely with life on any terms" (*TN* 30). Emmeline possesses (or is possessed by) "suspended" (*ibid.*, 49, 194) or "straying faculties" (*ibid.*, 125), perched in a state of "suspended crisis" like "one's last day on earth when fear and all sense of farewell had alike departed and only that very brief transit remained ahead" (*ibid.*, 140). And like Henry, she is stilled, a cheat of space and time:

> Her roll-top in its solemn surround of silence was a monument to the pretence of industry: in vain her stenographer's pointed tapping, in vain the clock: place and time, shivered to radiant atoms, were in disorder. There was no afternoon; the sun, forgetting decline, irresponsibly spun like a coin at the height of noonday. Emmeline, as though threatened with levitation, gripped the edge of her roll-top. (*Ibid.*, 118)

Like her property, Emmeline is "a monument to the pretence of industry", the pretence of mechanized life; suspended, "place and time" become atomized, "shivered", "disorder[ed]" – abstracted and meaningless.[21] Bennett and Royle see this as more broadly representative of space and time in Bowen, and argue that here, "What is fragmented or shivered is not only Emmeline's experience or state of mind: it is a shattering or shivering that can be seen to characterize any and every Bowenesque afternoon, or, more precisely, that haunts and thus conditions all 'place and time' in Bowen".[22] This underscores the juxtaposition of Emmeline with her clients, so that, as Maud Ellmann notes: "Emmeline moves by proxy while remaining at a standstill, static as the eye of a tornado."[23] However, this passage also suggests that Emmeline is engaged in a performance of normality ("I believe in façade", she claims [*TN* 24]), so that, as William Heath has

---

[21] Ellmann suggests that in *To the North*, "human beings become mechanical – spinning, twitching, shivering, and stilling, as if driven by remote control" (*The Shadow Across the Page*, 110). For Bennett and Royle the novel describes "the force of … going", a "radiance of atoms" (*Elizabeth Bowen and the Dissolution of the Novel*, 41).

[22] *Ibid.*, 31.

[23] Ellmann, *The Shadow Across the Page*, 103.

noted, her "dedication to the travel bureau, then, is her attempt to join vicariously in the experience of others, compensating for the psychological retreat she herself has made and for the passivity of her acquaintances".[24]

Under the "irresponsibl[e]" sun, the afternoon, temporal referent, ceases to have significance, while space is now so irrelevant that Emmeline may at any moment levitate. Moreover, the elements of hallucinatory psychosis in this passage foreshadow the closing moments of the novel, in which Emmeline speeds to her death: her desire for dissolution, for freedom from the pain of survival now at its height, Emmeline is no longer resistant to "levitation", or the "total loss of her faculties" (*TN* 244). Now, she "was lost to her own identity, a confining husk", while to Markie, her very "stillness" (*ibid.*, 242) figures a "remoteness that seemed more in time than in space" (*ibid.*, 244). This disregard for, or suspension outside of, temporality Emmeline elsewhere thinks of as the "air-mindedness" – "this distended present, this oppressive contraction of space would be properties of air-mindedness" – of the angel or the inhuman (*ibid.*, 144). It seems that more than resisting or rejecting temporality, Emmeline is unable to assimilate or to comprehend any time beyond the present. In Kristevan terms, this figuration of Emmeline as one for whom "time has been erased or bloated, absorbed into sorrow" reinforces her woundedness.[25] A state of spatial and temporal suspense thus comes to figure Emmeline's "retreat of thought" or "recoil" from life, and her movement towards dematerialization (*TN* 194).[26]

---

[24] Heath, "The Jacobean Melodrama of *To the North*", 28. See also Edwin J. Kenney, *Elizabeth Bowen*, London: Associated University Press, 1975, 42.

[25] Julia Kristeva, *Black Sun: Depression and Melancholia*, trans. Leon S. Roudiez, New York: Columbia University Press, 1989, 4. For Bennett and Royle, the "movement of time" in *To the North* "cannot be assimilated to the sensible or intelligible, to a commonsense perception of time as a continuous, homogeneous, linear unfolding or narrative" (*Elizabeth Bowen and the Dissolution of the Novel*, 26). Allan E. Austin argues that at the novel's conclusion, "Driving furiously, Emmeline seems determined to eclipse both time and space" (*Elizabeth Bowen*, Boston, MA: Twayne, 1989, 45). See also Jordan, *How Will the Heart Endure*, 67.

[26] Chris Hopkins has noted the confusion regarding selfhood in *To the North*, suggesting that its characters "worry about the fact that they do not seem to know what makes up their own selves" ("Elizabeth Bowen: Realism, Modernism and

Emmeline's psychic detachment is so heightened that even those around her appear to dissolve: she looks at Markie "as though he were not there" (*ibid.*, 72), and stares "so fixedly at Cecilia that Cecilia had disappeared" (*ibid.*, 98). Moreover, her psychic death so far precedes her physical dissolution that long before the novel's apocalyptic conclusion it is as if, for Cecilia, her sister-in-law does not exist:

> She looked into Emmeline's room, which, with counterpane drawn up over the pillow, looked shrouded, as though no one slept here now. A friend's room with its air of guarding a final secret is like a death-chamber; here, still unknown, the sleeper seems many times to have died ….
>
> Though the idea of parting from Emmeline could seem intolerable there was not much more, it occurred to Cecilia, than the idea of company in her company. Saying: "I live with Emmeline," she might paint for ignorant eyes, and even dazzle herself for a moment with a tempting picture of intimacy. But she lent herself to a fiction in which she did not believe; for she lived with nobody. (*Ibid.*, 132-33)

Emmeline is here at once dead, fictional, and nobody, her unreality repeated in simulacra which can only approximate to her estrangement from life. She "seems many times to have died", as each attempt to describe her non-existence further emphasizes her detachment. Emmeline, like Henry, is the ghost with whom Cecilia lies. Finally, that Cecilia "lived with nobody" underscores the fact that of the three Summers, she is the only survivor: Cecilia "live[s]", surrounded by "no body": the dead Henry and the falsely living Emmeline.

Death drives

Both *The Hotel* and *To the North* reach their climax during the "death drive" – Emmeline and Sydney's moments of traumatic recognition or assimilation. While in *To the North*, Emmeline's death might be read as a physical enactment of her psychological wound, in the earlier novel, the traumatic climax overlaps with the experience of the sublime, and enables Sydney's movement away from uncertainty and abjection, and towards a firmer sense of "aliveness". Indeed, LaCapra has noted that the sublime can itself be evoked by trauma, "by the

Gendered Identity in Her Novels of the 1930s", *Journal of Gender Studies*, IV/3 [1995], 272).

near-death experience, by coming to the brink of the abyss or of annihilation while escaping death and destruction oneself".[27] Importantly, both novels also link this moment of trauma to a disruption of the traditional female narrative plot. Early in *The Hotel*, Mrs Lee-Mittison, a guest at the eponymous residence, indulges in a private reverie. This dream constitutes two kinds of Modernist trauma: first, it figures the rural nostalgia common to writers of this period, but second, and perhaps more originally, the trauma of Bowen's novel describes the trauma or confusion of the seemingly inevitable female future, as the desire for the "bliss" of independence, of possessing rather than being possessed, of an "oasis of solitude", becomes unimaginable, even terrifying:

> Surprised at herself, she sat with bliss in her little oasis of solitude. She looked down the slope beside her into the valley below and saw a little house .... This little house which she seemed at once to inhabit gave her the most strange sensation of dignity and of peace. She saw herself go climbing up the garden from terrace to terrace, calling the goat, and the goat, beautiful in its possessedness, came loping down to meet her, asking to be milked. At this she paused in perplexity, for she had never milked anything and turned cold at the thought of touching the udders of an animal. But in a moment this was over and she carried the milk frothing warm in the pottery jug inside, into the dark interior of the house which would not be dark from within. Here something turned her back and she could not follow herself; she saddened, feeling excluded from some very intimate experience. The house was lonely and in autumn, when the river was brimming, the rushing past of the water must be terrifying .... The thud of a falling lemon would be enough to wake one in terror.
>
> The villino suddenly dropped away from her eye as though she had put down a telescope, and as her life sprang back into focus she must have been dizzy, for she felt sick at the thought of their hotel bedrooms that stretched, only interspersed with the spare-rooms of friends, in unbroken succession before and behind her. (*TH* 36-37)

Significantly, Mrs Lee-Mittison cannot cross the threshold of her fantasy, a liminal site which here moves from sublime pastoral bliss to

---

[27] Dominick LaCapra, *History and Memory after Auschwitz*, Ithaca, NY: Cornell University Press, 1998, 35. LaCapra here refers to ideas expressed by Immanuel Kant in *The Critique of Judgment* (1790).

those traumatic and repetitive "thud[s]" of terror. It is then with dizziness, a sense of vertigo – perched on the brink of the abyss – that she returns to reality, to dependence, to uncertain rootlessness, to the disappointment of the expected narrative of marriage, anticipating, in fact, the life of the Montmorencys in Bowen's next novel, *The Last September*. In Bowen's early fiction, this current of personal, specifically female, trauma, gains importance through its juxtaposition with, and underscoring of, the broader political and cultural trauma of the interwar period.

Bowen's first novel is often compared to Virginia Woolf's *The Voyage Out* (1915), to the work of E.M. Forster, and of Henry James, and concerns the activities and conversations of guests spending a winter on the Italian Riviera.[28] Sydney Warren, the novel's protagonist (if she can be called that, for she does so little), a "probable twenty-two" and a medical student, has been sent away on a holiday with her elder cousin Tessa by her relations, who fear that the stress of Sydney's recent examinations may lead to a "breakdown" (*TH* 11, 17). During her stay, Sydney becomes devoted to Mrs Kerr, a widow in her forties – the first of the recurring manipulative elder women in Bowen's fiction.[29] However, the arrival of the clergyman, James Milton, and then of Mrs Kerr's son, Ronald, disrupts the careful routine of the hotel. On her son's arrival, Mrs Kerr drops Sydney and shifts her attention to him; Sydney, shocked by this abandonment, seeks company in Milton and, almost accidentally, becomes engaged to him. The dramatic drive back from a hotel excursion jolts Sydney into what may be called an awakening to, or a recognition of, life, but certainly into the realization that she does not wish to marry Milton. She calls off their engagement, whereupon Milton and Ronald, who no longer "matter", leave the hotel (*ibid.*, 81). The novel concludes where it had started, circling back, through the recollections of Miss Pym and Miss Fitzgerald, to the feud from which it set out. As

[28] See, for example, Lee, *Elizabeth Bowen*, 59; Neil Corcoran, *Elizabeth Bowen: The Enforced Return*, Oxford: Oxford University Press, 2004, 4. Coates even excludes *The Hotel* from his study of Bowen's novels because, he states, "the work is derivative" (*Social Discontinuity in the Novels of Elizabeth Bowen*, 7).

[29] Specifically, I refer to Lady Naylor in *The Last September*, Lady Waters in *To the North*, Lady Elfrida in *Friends and Relations*, Mme Fisher in *The House in Paris*, and Antonia in *A World of Love*, as well as numerous others in Bowen's short fiction.

Ellmann has so neatly pointed out, the entire narrative of *The Hotel* occurs within the wound of the rift opened up by this couple.[30]

Like Emmeline in *To the North*, Sydney suffers from an inability to engage in life, a kind of nothingness of the self. Yet, while Bowen's later heroine is in what seems to be a permanent state of detachment that foreshadows her ultimate death, Sydney, on the other hand, appears to balance on the brink of this kind of impassiveness. Although she is repeatedly described as "strange" (*TH* 20, 60, 62, 141), "remote" (*ibid.*, 1), "detach[ed]" (*ibid.*, 82), "out of place" (*ibid.*, 27), "a little out of time" (*ibid.*, 29), and although this is underscored by the suggestion that the hotel, site of transience, is a "doll's house" (*ibid.*, 68), there is, in this novel, an uncertainty regarding the degree of Sydney's estrangement. That is, while Emmeline enforces her own detachment, certain that "no one could [locate] me, and no one seems to expect me to do it for them" (*TN* 192), Sydney makes her existence dependent on others – and in particular, Mrs Kerr:

> If she did not exist for Mrs Kerr as a tennis player, in this most ordinary, popular of her aspects, had she reason to feel she existed at all? It became no longer a question of – What did Mrs Kerr think of her? – but rather – Did Mrs Kerr ever think of her? The possibility of not being kept in mind seemed to Sydney at that moment a kind of extinction. (*TH* 14)

It is this sense of being cast out, or expelled from Mrs Kerr, "of not being kept in mind", which impels in Sydney "a kind of extinction" – a state more permanent, more absolute, than death, suggesting a complete erasure of life, and the impossibility of return. What is so horrific in this passage is Sydney's traumatic recognition that she appears at once present – in the betrayal of her self-centredness, a hyper self-awareness – and obliterated: it is not, in fact, Mrs Kerr who consigns her to "extinction", but Sydney who thinks herself into non-entity, into the very impossibility of thought.[31] This is complicated, however, by Sydney's additional uncertainty about the reality or

---

[30] Ellmann, *The Shadow Across the Page*, 74.

[31] "Rather than thinking themselves", suggest Bennett and Royle, "people in Bowen are … *being thought*" (*Elizabeth Bowen and the Dissolution of the Novel*, 9; original emphasis).

existence of others, those on whom she relies for the perception of her own existence:

> She was accustomed to stare at people as from a point of vantage, forgetting she too had a face. They had thoughts, too (with these she often forgot to credit them); did *they* also think as they looked at oneself? (*TH* 17; original emphasis)

Identity, for Sydney, is always held in suspense, on the threshold, on the brink, foreshadowing the novel's climactic drive on the edge of the abyss. Thus, Sydney is at once existent and non-existent, a figure of abjection. She is simultaneously the abject thing of horror and caught in terrified reaction to this traumatic collapse of her identity, the breakdown in meaning the abject represents.

Sydney's engagement to Milton arises from a desire to survive – to escape this abjection. It is only after conversations with other women in the hotel and in particular with Veronica, another young guest, in which her friend wonders, "Does it ever occur to you that being alive is a mistake?" and demands "But what am *I* to do? I don't want to *be* anything .... Tell me what you think will become of me", that Sydney accepts Milton's proposal (*ibid.*, 97, 99; original emphasis). Veronica alerts Sydney to the idea that the female condition of "being" is impossible without adhering to the traditional narrative plot of marriage: "Everybody's the same and I must have somebody" (*ibid.*, 99).[32] Sydney also overhears a circle of married women, one of whom observes:

> "As winter comes on with those long evenings one begins to feel hardly human, sitting evening after evening in an empty room .... If I shut my drawing-room door, I begin to feel restless at once; it feels so unnatural shutting oneself in with nobody .... It's not, of course, that I'm nervous, but I really begin to feel – if you'll understand my saying anything so extraordinary – as if I didn't exist. If somebody does

---

[32] Andrew Bennett has observed that Bowen's "early novels are focused unerringly on young women and concern their post-war resistance to the teleology of the marriage plot ... and the related concern that romantic love is no longer possible or viable, or the solution to the condition of being a woman, is the fundamental crisis of Bowen's early, Modernist fiction" ("Bowen and Modernism: The Early Novels", in *Elizabeth Bowen*, ed. Eibhear Walshe, Dublin: Irish Academic Press, 2009, 29-30). See also Jordan, *How Will the Heart Endure*, 39-40.

> come to the door or the telephone does ring, I'm almost surprised to find I'm still there. One would go mad if one were not able to get abroad."
>
> She looked round with a shiver of retrospection at the semi-circle which was her pleasant asylum .... What they had all escaped was terrible. (*TH* 53-54)

It is through one's relationship with others, Sydney learns from the other women at the hotel, that one overcomes this nothingness of the self, "sitting evening after evening" in an empty room. Yet implicit here is that the abyss from which these women have only just "escaped" is not just a routine at home, but something worse: the permanent nonexistence of the unmarried woman. It is possible, then, that Sydney sees Milton as a ("business-like" [*ibid.*, 126]) solution to her abjection: her engagement will place her in a position of certainty, and give her an existence in relation to another, an identity within society. The novel's climactic "death drive", however, jolts Sydney into a recognition of her existence without these dependencies, so that this moment of trauma works simultaneously as a moment of sublime release into true survival.

The experiences of trauma and of the sublime, Frank Ankersmit has noted, are both characterized by dissociation, and provoke detachment as a coping mechanism:

> The subject of a traumatic experience is peculiarly numbed by it; he is, so to speak, put at a distance from what caused it. The traumatic experience is dissociated from one's "normal" experience of the world .... [In the tranquil experience of the sublime] we have distanced ourselves from a situation of *real* danger – and in this way, we have *dissociated* ourselves from the object of experience. The sublime thus provokes a movement of derealization by which reality is robbed of its threatening potentialities.[33]

LaCapra, too, notes that the connection between trauma and the sublime involves three components: "a rupture or blockage of some sort (for example, of understanding); a flooding of the system or potentially traumatizing excess (for example, of anxiety, terror ...);

[33] Frank Ankersmit, *Sublime Historical Experience*, Stanford, CA: Stanford University Press, 2005, 335-36 (original emphasis).

and elation (for example, at surviving the risk of rupture and excess)."[34] Sydney exhibits all of these during the treacherous drive of the novel's climax: not only is her relationship with Mrs Kerr definitively ruptured immediately preceding the drive, she appears to suffer a "blockage" in terms of her inability to think or to imagine a future with Milton ("Such a little slip of a thing … I don't think she *understands*", Mrs Lee-Mittison had already observed of the engagement [*TH* 124]).[35]

The "violent" and terrifying excess of the drive down the mountain, a drive "not like motoring at all", but "more like *dropping*", is a moment of abject trauma that reveals the ever-present possibility of death. This then gives way, in Sydney, to an intense sense of clarity:

> She sat back quietly and began to concentrate her whole will and imagination. "If it could be the next corner," she thought, "we should go over clean – there is that clear drop. Let it be the next corner ..." But the next corner was past. The rush of air and the movement had made her come alive again and she seemed to herself to be reasoning very clearly and accurately.
>
> … Her mind became quite quiet again and she went on saying. "The next corner ... the *next* corner."
>
> Round the next, barely round it, the brakes jarred, the car swayed on locked wheels and stopped dead. (*TH* 156-57; original emphasis)

The detachment demonstrated by Sydney throughout the novel is here at the height of derealization or the refusal of danger, as she "began to be perfectly sure of what was coming, perfectly confident". At this simultaneous moment of trauma and of the sublime, the abjection of fear and of *jouissance*, Sydney suddenly "come[s] alive again" (*ibid.*, 157), and (in metaphors which conjure this combination of the knowledge of death and exhilaration of life), "for the first time felt life sharply, life as keen as death to bite upon the consciousness, pressed

[34] LaCapra, *History and Memory*, 33-34.

[35] Ellmann recognizes that "Sydney, who suffers from 'a strange anaesthesia', could be seen as a living embodiment of impasse, blocked from without and from within" (*The Shadow Across the Page*, 71).

inexorably upon her, held to her throat like a knife" (*ibid.*, 158).[36] It is at this point that Sydney moves from being "as inanimate and objective as a young girl in a story told by a man, incapable of a thought or a feeling that was not attributed to her, with no personality of her own", to being a woman in her own story (*TH* 156).

Sydney becomes the author and protagonist of her own narrative, but more significantly, the trauma or disruption of the male plot makes way for the sublime, the *jouissance*, of female narrative. The way in which the sublime enables this "non-decision", and allows the novel to "resist the narrative of romantic love", in Andrew Bennett's words, might then go some way to answering Ellman's question: "And how can the novel, which traditionally ends in death or marriage, accommodate itself to women's new and unpredictable trajectories?"[37] This "new and unpredictable" trajectory is made literal in *The Hotel* in Sydney's "death drive", for it is at the point at which Sydney wishes for, and hovers on the brink of, destruction, the moment which figures a traumatic recognition of the wounded self, that the expected female narrative trajectory is disrupted. The experience of the sublime thus removes Sydney from suspension and from dependent identity; in "the shock of being alive", the realization that "we were as real as this", Sydney is no longer a marionette, or a character in another's plot (*TH* 160). As in no other Bowen novel, in *The Hotel*, the experience of trauma does not wound but, in its overlap with the sublime, functions as a restorative. Sydney's survival is precisely a condition of her trauma.

---

[36] Ellmann and Lee both use metaphors of sleep and waking to describe the change in Sydney (Ellmann, *The Shadow Across the Page*, 76; Lee, *Elizabeth Bowen*, 59).

[37] Bennett, "Bowen and Modernism", 27, 32; Ellmann, *The Shadow Across the Page*, 70.

CHAPTER 2

SUPPLEMENT: *THE LAST SEPTEMBER*

> But the supplement supplements. It adds only to replace. It intervenes or insinuates itself in-the-place-of; if it fills, it is as one fills a void. If it represents and makes an image, it is by the anterior default of a presence. Compensatory [*suppléant*] and vicarious, the supplement is an adjunct, a subaltern instance which takes-(the)-place [*tient-lieu*]. As substitute, it is not simply added to the positivity of a presence, it produces no relief, its place is assigned in the structure by the mark of an emptiness. Somewhere, something can be filled up of itself, can accomplish itself, only by allowing itself to be filled through sign and proxy. The sign is always the supplement of the thing itself.[1]

> Meanwhile Lois was very melancholy in the box-room …. On the whitewash, her mother, to whom also the box-room had been familiar, had written L.N., L.N., and left an insulting drawing of somebody, probably Hugo. She had scrawled with passion; she had never been able to draw. Lois looked and strained after feeling, but felt nothing.[2]

The Last September is a novel structured by the supplementary – by addition, inscription, construction, invasion. These supplements are underpinned by "the mark of an emptiness", the absent thing "filled through sign and proxy". Indeed, it is as if the narrative (the sign) is shadowed or haunted by that for which it is supplement, "the thing itself". Phyllis Lassner and Neil Corcoran, most notably, have

---

[1] Jacques Derrida, "... That Dangerous Supplement ..." (1967), trans. Gayatri Chakravorty Spivak (1976), in *Acts of Literature*, ed. Derek Attridge, New York: Routledge, 1992, 83.
[2] Elizabeth Bowen, *The Last September* (1929), New York: Anchor, 2000, 192. Hereafter cited parenthetically as *LS*.

recognized the "lack" which describes Bowen's second novel.[3] These ideas about lack and supplementarity inform a reading of trauma inscribed on, and inscribed in, space: the ruined mill and Danielstown's box-room. The architecture of Danielstown mimics the architecture of the traumatized psyche in which trauma, in Freud's terms, is repressed, and according to Abraham and Torok, is encrypted or entombed, in the psychological topography.[4] The box-room, in which the long-dead Laura Naylor is memorialized by the inscriptions she has left on its walls, figures the absent presence – the lack and the supplement – of traumatic memory. Writing and the storehouse are both obvious metaphors for memory, and these textual remains work to memorialize – indeed, to immortalize – Laura. The absent Laura is made present, made to survive, through these scrawls, for the sign and the memorial work in similar ways to supplement a lack, to "take-(the)-place", to hold the place of, "the thing itself". This reading of the architecture of trauma in *The Last September* is elaborated by an examination of Danielstown's "Other", the horrific ruined mill.[5] The abjection of the ruin at once figures the maintenance and the disruption of spatial and temporal continuity, and works as a site of trauma in the narrative, in the landscape, and in the novel's sense of an Anglo-Irish heritage.

Much like Bowen's first novel, *The Hotel*, *The Last September* is concerned with the difficulties of adolescent female identity. However, as critics have argued, in the later novel the uncertainties of nineteen-year-old Lois Farquar are more clearly tied to those of post-First World War Europe, and in particular, of Ireland and the Anglo-

---

[3] Phyllis Lassner, "The Past Is a Burning Pattern: Elizabeth Bowen's *The Last September*", *Eire-Ireland*, XXI/1 (Spring 1986), 43; Neil Corcoran, "Discovery of a Lack: History and Ellipsis in Elizabeth Bowen's *The Last September*", *Irish University Review*, XXXII/2 (Autumn-Winter 2001), 315.

[4] See Sigmund Freud, "Beyond the Pleasure Principle" (1920), in *The Essentials of Psycho-Analysis*, ed. Anna Freud, trans. James Strachey, London: Vintage, 2005, 223, 228; Nicolas Abraham and Maria Torok, "The Topography of Reality: Sketching a Metapsychology of Secrets" (1971), in *The Shell and the Kernel: Renewals of Psychoanalysis*, trans. Nicholas T. Rand, Chicago, IL: University of Chicago Press, 1994, I, 159.

[5] Corcoran has similarly argued that the mill is Danielstown's dark Other ("Discovery of a Lack", 329).

Irish during the Troubles.[6] The threshold existence of the adolescent girl becomes a figure, in this novel, for national and international political uncertainty in 1920s Ireland.

The Last September is the first of Bowen's novels to adopt what will become a familiar tripartite structure, and the subtitles of the three sections – "The Arrival of the Montmorencys", "The Visit of Miss Norton", and "The Departure of Gerald" – pick up on the hospitality intrinsic to the Big House. The novel's first section works to reinforce the established way of life of the Anglo-Irish gentry – the daily visits, tennis parties, and scheduled lunches which demarcate the regularity and routine of Danielstown, and households like it. There is, nevertheless, an underlying sense of unease about the political turmoil in the region. Upon their arrival, for example, the Montmorencys are immediately asked if there had been "trouble" on their journey, though this is just as quickly covered by questions about tea (*LS* 4). That insidious disquiet foreshadows the more explicit violence of the novel's concluding scenes. But it is Lois' self-conscious desire for romantic love which is foregrounded, and this is, at this stage, focused on the much older Hugo Montmorency, whom she recalls visiting her mother (to whom he was once engaged) several years previously.

This infatuation is disrupted by the arrival of Marda Norton in the novel's second section. Marda exemplifies a modern femininity to which Lois aspires and her passion for Marda approaches homosexual desire. Indeed, it is after Lois and Marda's most intimate encounter – their visit to the ruined mill and discovery there of an Irish rebel – that Lois decides upon the "safety" of marriage to Gerald Lesworth, a young British lieutenant. The novel's third section links the personal and political plots as the growing violence across the countryside enters the domestic realm. It is in this final section that Gerald does, in effect, depart twice over: Lois and Gerald's engagement is swiftly dissolved by the disapproving Lady Naylor, and shortly after that, Gerald is killed while on patrol. Lois, too, has left Danielstown prior to the novel's apocalyptic conclusion. Her going away repeats Laura's earlier departure from the Big House or, perhaps, Laura's departure anticipates her daughter's. Laura's never-told narrative forms a

[6] See Jordan, *How Will the Heart Endure*, 48; Kenney, *Elizabeth Bowen*, 33; Lassner, "The Past is a Burning Pattern", 48; Heather Ingman, *Twentieth-Century Fiction by Irish Women: Nation and Gender*, Aldershot: Ashgate, 2007, 32-33.

traumatic absence which Lois' plot supplements; Lois is the supplement for Laura. Laura is survived by Lois, but Lois is shadowed by the lost mother.

The temporal structures of *The Last September* complicate this condition of anticipation or, more specifically, anxiety (the anticipation of trauma) in the narrative. Jed Esty, for example, notes that the Anglo-Irish of *The Last September* are "an extinction waiting to happen", and points out that the "odd temporality of anticipated doom in the novel's 1920 setting – combined with the retrospective foreclosure of its 1928-9 date of composition" is mirrored by Lois, "the living figure of a cultural death".[7] *The Last September*, Bowen later wrote, was the only one of her novels

> … to be set back deliberately, in a former time …. "All this," I willed the reader to know, "is done with and over". From the start, the reader must look, be conscious of looking, backward – down a backward perspective of eight years.[8]

This "backward perspective" means that the personal and the political plots of *The Last September* anticipate traumas that have always already happened. Thus Francie has "very strongly a sense of return" (*LS* 14) since Danielstown is already razed, its inhabitants already dead or departed, the story already at its culminating "blank full stop" even before it has begun (*ibid.*, 53). If Freud's *Angstbereitschaft*, anxiety-preparedness, figures a learned desire not to be caught unaware by trauma, then it follows that a condition of anxiety is contingent upon an awareness of the aversive future.[9] That is, even as it arises as a consequence of a traumatic past, "dreading forward" to the traumatic event is always and everywhere dependent upon progression towards the time when that event will occur.[10] The

---

[7] Jed Esty, "Virgins of Empire: *The Last September* and the Antidevelopmental Plot", *Modern Fiction Studies*, LII/3 (Summer 2007), 271.

[8] Elizabeth Bowen, "Preface to *The Last September*", 124.

[9] If, Freud notes, "The present situation reminds me of one of the traumatic experiences I have had before … I will anticipate the trauma and behave as though it had already come, while there is yet time to turn aside" ("Inhibitions, Symptoms and Anxiety" [1926], in *The Standard Edition of the Complete Psychological Works of Sigmund Freud*, London: Hogarth, 1953-73, XX, 166).

[10] Lyndsey Stonebridge, *The Writing of Anxiety: Imagining Wartime in Mid-Century British Culture*, Houndmills: Palgrave Macmillan, 2007, 6.

complicated temporality of *The Last September* thus exposes the ways in which the anticipation and the recollection of trauma work, so that in the experience of anxiety we also experience traumatic recall. It is in this conflict between anticipation and retrospection that *The Last September* has the most to say about trauma, its expectation and its recollection, and about the ways in which trauma disrupts the configuration of linear temporality.

This temporal disruption is underpinned by the novel's emphasis on the atemporality or stasis of the Anglo-Irish, on their spatial isolation – the house and its inhabitants are "enisled" – and on their refusal to acknowledge the future in the form of the growing political threat (*LS* 28). Even when the Black and Tans return Laurence's stolen watch, still ticking, the Naylors fail to read this as a threat, as the countdown to Danielstown's destruction (*ibid.*, 278). It seems that the Anglo-Irish of *The Last September* exist in a perfect present – that frozen "moment of happiness, of perfection" on which the novel opens (*ibid.*, 3). Even Lois, who is so impatient for the future that it is as if she is "being driven against time to catch a train" (*ibid.*, 118), is helpless, paralysed, "cocoon[ed]" (*ibid.*, 66) by social expectation, and "keeps hearing that final train go out without her" (*ibid.*, 118).[11] This suspension of time means that *The Last September* exists in something like Lois' "ideal no-place" (*LS* 127), or in that vacuum created by all the novel's yawns (*ibid.*, 5, 58, 86, 116, 135). To locate a sense of anticipation in the novel is difficult precisely because of this refusal of the novel's Anglo-Irish to imagine or acknowledge futurity; their rejection of the future is a defence mechanism, not only against the traumatic future, but against even preparedness for it. The behaviour of the Naylors and their guests is a defence doubled: a defence against the need for defence.[12]

---

[11] For Lee, it is Lois' very "impatience" which "anticipates the tragic destruction of the house", as "Her desire to be violently precipitated into her future is granted with a vengeance: it's as though her restlessness partly *wills* the end of Danielstown" (*Elizabeth Bowen*, 48; original emphasis).

[12] See also Maria DiBattista, who argues that traumatic events like Gerald's death are not anticipated by the residents of Danielstown because the "patterns of country life, its rounds of arrivals and departures, help dispel the very anxiety that would have helped the besieged community to anticipate and so possibly circumvent such violent departures", and that "if Irish history is a nightmare from which Bowen's novel is trying to awake, it conforms to the classic Freudian description of the anxiety dream,

It is in recoil from this "blank full stop" of the "confrontation of a positive futurelessness", that Laurence, would-be novelist, rewrites the narrative's history:

> ... his mind ran spiderlike back on the thread spun out of itself for advance, stumbling and swerving a little over its own intricacy. He caught trains he had missed, rushing out to the boundless possible through the shining mouths of termini, re-ordered meals in a cosmopolitan blur, re-ate them, thought of thought but sheered away from that windy gulf full of a fateful clapping of empty book-covers. Far enough back, in a kind of unborn freedom, he even remade marriages .... Here, in this that had been her room, Laura had lain on her wedding morning, watching a spider run up to the canopy of the bed ... Laurence, to be acclaimed a second Weiniger, blew out his brains at – say – Avila, in a fit of temporary discouragement without having heard of Danielstown. Lois, naturally, was not born at all. (*LS* 153-54)

In ways that foreshadow Bowen's next novel, *Friends and Relations*, *The Last September* is thus ghosted by what Corcoran has called "a kind of plot unconscious".[13] This alternative narrative plot is a means by which Laurence works to expose the novel's voids, and to replace the supplement with that which it hides, the "thing itself" – with Laura's narrative, no longer over but now "still impending" (*LS* 154). It is worth noting that Laurence's reverie is precipitated by the disappointing absence of raiders outside his window: "there were no bicycles; no one knocked; all he had to say went sour in him" (*ibid.*, 153). It is in response to this nothingness, to this "sour" decay, that Laurence writes himself (and, indeed, Lois), the supplements, out of existence, in what Corcoran calls a "dissolving oneiric vision" that makes way for the novel's spectre, Laura.[14] Yet, like Lois, for whom "not to be known of seemed like a doom of extinction" (*LS* 42), and like Sydney in *The Hotel*, for whom "[t]he possibility of not being

---

in which traumatic events are felt to have been insufficiently anticipated" ("Elizabeth Bowen's Troubled Modernism", in *Modernism and Colonialism: British and Irish Literature, 1899-1939*, eds Richard Begam and Michael Valdez Moses, Durham, NC: Duke University Press, 2007, 237).

[13] Corcoran, "Discovery of a Lack", 318. See also my discussion of the spectral plots of *Friends and Relations* in Chapter 3.

[14] *Ibid.*, 317.

kept in mind seemed … a kind of extinction" (*TH* 14), it is impossible for Laurence not to keep himself in Laura's mind; that is, to think the trauma of his own extinction. His figuration of his thought, of himself as "spiderlike", therefore exists even in the alternative plot he spins: Laurence is the spider, watched by the resurrected bride, Laura.

But Laurence is not the only one to create this kind of supplementary narrative. Hugo authors an alternative narrative plot in which, avoiding the futurelessness and passivity of his nomadic life with Francie, he can act on his love for Marda: "he seemed to have stepped through into some kind of non-existence … divorced equally from fact and from probability, he set up a stage for himself" (*LS* 259).[15] And when Lois arrives at a traumatic recognition of the futurelessness that would describe her potential marriage to Gerald, she too escapes into spatial absence, "nonentity", an "ideal no-place":

> So that was being kissed: just an impact, with inside blankness. She was lonely, and saw there was no future. She shut her eyes and tried … to be enclosed in nonentity, in some ideal no-place perfect and clear as a bubble. (*LS* 127)

When she writes to Marda of this (non-)future with Gerald, Lois is, like Laurence, halted by that "blank full stop":

> But as a matter of fact, I have no future, in their sense. I have promised to marry Gerald.
>
> Here she paused, for from now on it was all obscure ahead of her. … But when she looked for Gerald there seemed too much of him. He was a wood in which she counted from tree to tree – all hers – and knew the boundary wall right round. But how to measure this unaccountable darkness between the trees, this living silence? (*Ibid.*, 258-59)

If it is true, as Derrida asserts, that the supplement "is maddening because it is neither presence nor absence", then what Lois has

[15] Hugo is characterized by this "way of avoiding things" (*LS* 166); in Ellmann's words, he "wallows in his disappointments: the woman he never married, the move to Canada he never risked, the bungalow he never bought, the furniture that will never be unstored" (*The Shadow Across the Page*, 61).

recognized is precisely this "maddening" unaccountability in Gerald, neither presence nor absence, neither the wood nor the darkness.[16] Gerald Lesworth is un(ac)countable because he is at once "worthless" (in the sense that he is, finally, nothing to Lois), and "too much" (in the sense that he overwhelms Lois with his desire for her). Moreover, Gerald insists upon supplementing Lois with his own idea of her, an idea "inaccessible to her; she could not affect it" (*LS* 65); he kisses only "the thought of [her]" (*ibid.*, 238) and she is, for him, a poultice (or supplement) for "this ache, this absence" (*ibid.*, 126). This means that just as Lois is unable to account for Gerald, he also fails to read or to account for her, as she recognizes when she laments:

> "I feel certain you have illusions about me, I don't believe you know what I'm like a bit." And while she spoke she counted the crimson strings in her racquet: three down, six across. (*Ibid.*, 60)[17]

Here, too, what is present – "the crimson strings" – can be counted, while the spaces between those strings, equally important to the racquet's construction, form an unaccountable and uncounted "darkness". As the last sentence of this chapter, that darkness stretches across the textual vacancy until the narrative resumes. This "unaccountable darkness" is also produced in Lois' response to overhearing Francie about to "stop, seal, finish" her in definition: an act of violence which produces a crack in her bedroom basin, "running between a sheaf and a cornucopia: a harvest richness to which she each day bent down her face" (*ibid.*, 83). As when Lois bids goodbye to Marda through a crack in the door (*ibid.*, 202), to later see or speak through that crack – what Carmen Concilio describes as a "gap in the discourse" – and wonder "what Lois *was*" (*ibid.*, 83; original emphasis) is to recognize, again, the importance of the void or the darkness when accounting for identity.[18]

---

[16] Derrida, "That Dangerous Supplement", 96. In these instances Bowen also argues for narrative as a shadowed supplement, and thus the condition of secrecy in the "ideal literary object", which I will develop in Chapter 8.

[17] Francie, too, has illusions about Lois' identity, the girl recognizes, when she "feel[s] the bright girl she had been for Mrs Montmorency disintegrate: much that even she had taken to be herself went with the illusion" (*LS* 275).

[18] Carmen Concilio, "Things That Do Speak in Elizabeth Bowen's *The Last September*", in *Moments of Moment: Aspects of the Literary Epiphany*, ed. Wim

That darkness also becomes what is unaccounted for by the Naylors, the growing threat that they refuse to acknowledge. In this second use of the metaphor of the forest and the darkness in *The Last September*, the insidious dusk again blurs the boundaries of certainty:

> Looking down, it seemed to Lois they lived in a forest; space of lawns blotted out in the pressure and dusk of trees. She wondered they were not smothered; then wondered still more that they were not afraid .... Only the massed trees – spread like a rug to dull some keenness, break some contact between self and senses perilous to the routine of living – only the trees of the demesne were dark and exhaled darkness .... Dusk would lie where one looked as though it were in one's eyes, as though the fountain of darkness were in one's own perception. Seen from above, the house in its pit of trees seemed a very reservoir of obscurity; from the doors one must come out stained with it. (*LS* 92-93)

Danielstown is not characterized by the safety of "home"; rather, the Big House is hidden in, and "blotted out" by, the darkness, the "pressure and dusk" of the "massed trees". Indeed, it is this inability to distinguish the trees from the darkness in this passage that is most disturbing, for even as the trees work to "dull" or numb the "senses" to a "keenness ... perilous to the routine of living" – in order to "live how one can" – the house and its residents are "smothered" by and incorporated into the surrounding darkness. (Recall that for Laurence, this infiltration of dusk figures the very futurelessness from which he retreats, as night falls and the darkness resumes "with an uncomfortable suggestion of normality" [*ibid.*, 153].) Moreover, as they choke or drown in the dusk, the residents of Danielstown are forced to gulp in the "fountain of darkness", to incorporate it, inescapably, into themselves, to be "stained" with that very gap in their discourse, the threatening absent presence they refuse to name: the silenced Other that is the subaltern Irish culture.[19]

Tigges, Amsterdam: Rodopi, 1999, 287. For Lassner, "The effect of being talked about instead of spoken to, of overhearing directly the determination of one's fate, is to diminish the sense of a living self" (*Elizabeth Bowen*, 36).

[19] Seamus Deane asserts that in Irish literature written in English between 1880 and 1950 can be heard the "tragic ... silence of the other language that haunts the English language" ("Dumbness and Eloquence: A Note on English as We Write It in Ireland", in *Ireland and Postcolonial Theory*, eds Clare Carroll and Patricia King, Notre Dame,

This penetration of the structure and safety of the domestic by the threatening Other of "outside" represents a traumatic collapse of that familiar dichotomy of inside and outside (culture and nature) described by Gaston Bachelard.[20] It is in this overwhelming of the inside by the outside, the light of culture and modernity by the darkness of nature and the primitive – that is, the infiltration of the Self by the Other – that Danielstown approaches a fate already figured in the text: that of the ruined mill. Indeed, Danielstown is not only "smothered" by the dark trees, but substituted by the mill itself, and thus supplemented by the dark Other. Moreover, insofar as the mill is the hiding-place for the gunman Lois and Marda disturb, this ruin also functions as the site at which darkness, Otherness, and Irish rebellion coincide. This forced entry of the outside, of darkness, and of the Other therefore figures a symbolic eviction of the Naylors by the Irish rebels, even before the novel's final conflagration.

This slippage between inside and outside, the collapse of boundaries, figures the traumatic abjection of the ruin, in which, Dylan Trigg notes, "You are still *inside*. It is not that you have made it outside but that *the outside has made its way in*."[21] It is that abjection, the horrific decay of the "Incredible" "corpse" of the mill which induces terror in Lois:

> "Oh, what *is* that? The ghost of a Palace Hotel?"
>
> The mill startled them all, staring light-eyed, ghoulishly, round a bend of the valley. Lois had to come hurrying up to explain how it frightened her. In fact she wouldn't for worlds go into it but liked going as near as she dared. It was a fear she didn't want to get over, a kind of deliciousness. These dead mills – the country was full of them, never quite stripped and whitened to skeleton's decency: like corpses

---

IN: University of Notre Dame Press, 2003, 119). The traumatic voids of adolescent and Anglo-Irish identity then here expand to take in the postcolonial implications of the novel. Beth Wightman, too, recognizes the way in which the presence of "Irish islandness … figured here as the IRA", threatens to overwhelm what she sees as the "absence" of Anglo-Irish identity ("Geopolitics and the Sight of the Nation: Elizabeth Bowen's *The Last September*", *LIT*, XVIII/1 [Jan-Mar 2007], 51, 57).

[20] Gaston Bachelard, *The Poetics of Space*, trans. Maria Jolas (1958), Boston: Beacon, 1964. For Concilio, the threat of "out there" is also a function of the novel's postcolonialism ("Things That Do Speak", 286).

[21] Dylan Trigg, *The Aesthetics of Decay: Nothingness, Nostalgia, and the Absence of Reason*, ed. Robert Ginsberg, New York: Peter Lang, 2006, 249 (original emphasis).

> at their most horrible. "Another," Hugo declared, "of our national grievances. English law strangled the –" ….
>
> The river darkened and thundered towards the millrace, light came full on the high façade of decay. Incredible in its loneliness, roofless, floorless, beams criss-crossing the dank interior daylight, the whole place tottered, fit to crash at a breath. Hinges rustily bled where a door had been wrenched away; up six storeys panes still tattered the daylight …. the dead mill now entered the democracy of ghostliness, equalled broken palaces in futility and sadness; was transfigured by some response of the spirit, showing not the decline of its meanness, simply decline; took on all of a past to which it had given nothing. (*LS* 178-79; original emphasis)

The mill's horrifying abjection and its attendant terror is not only a function of its "bleeding" hinges and its corpse-like qualities, but of its temporal disruption. Indeed, the ruin for Trigg is "an object that, while still persisting in space and time, is displaced from its narrative context and so points to an elsewhere that is no longer".[22] Several critics have explored the significance of the mill in terms of *The Last September*'s engagement with cultural and historical forces, as well as its role in the development of Lois' female (and sexual) identity.[23] Yet, what remains to be discussed are those ways in which the figure of the ruin, what Trigg terms "traumatized architecture", contributes to an exploration of Bowen's writing of trauma.[24] In particular, such a reading disrupts the architectural memorialization and monumentalization represented by, for example, *Bowen's Court*.[25]

---

[22] *Ibid.*, 29. A similar horror afflicts the narrator of Edgar Allan Poe's "The Fall of the House of Usher" (1839), an architectural debt acknowledged in *The Last September* (*LS* 180).

[23] See, for example, Corcoran, "Discovery of a Lack", 326-29; Lassner, "The Past is a Burning Pattern", 51; C.L. Innes, "Custom, Ceremony and Innocence: Elizabeth Bowen's *The Last September*", in *Troubled Histories, Troubled Fictions: Twentieth-Century Anglo-Irish Prose*, eds Theo D'haen and José Lanters, Amsterdam: Rodopi, 1995, 108; Ann Owens Weekes, *Irish Women Writers: An Uncharted Tradition*, Lexington: University Press of Kentucky, 1990, 100-102; Ellen M. Wolff, *"An Anarchy in the Mind and in the Heart": Narrating Anglo-Ireland*, Harrisburg, PA: Bucknell University Press, 2006, 97-98.

[24] Dylan Trigg, "The Place of Trauma: Memory, Hauntings, and the Temporality of Ruins", *Memory Studies*, II/1 (January 2009), 94.

[25] In Bowen's description of the architecture of Bowen's Court in her family memoir, she maintains the present tense because, she says, "*I* saw no reason to transpose it into

The untimely ruin figures the strange temporality of decay, as the architectural corpse both recalls and destroys its traumatic past – a trauma which is thus always already present.[26] In this way, the ruin holds trauma in suspense, as the liminal state of decay means that the structure is never quite dead, and is held in the spatial and temporal indeterminacy of ghostliness, of the hanging strangulation of Hugo's unfinished sentence.[27] What is striking is that Lois mimics that suspense when she approaches the mill, not only holding her fear in abeyance, but appearing to hold her breath for fear of the ruin's collapse (*LS* 179). Before the ruin, Lois mirrors the mill's tension, compelled to bear witness to the continuing event of trauma it audaciously displays.

Just as the silences in a text point to the impossibility of representing trauma, the unspeakable limit-event, so too the cracks and crevasses of the ruin figure the unrepresentable.[28] Furthermore, the traumatized structure of the ruin itself forms a cleft in the landscape not unlike the absent presence of traumatic memory in the human psyche.[29] In this way, Corcoran argues, the mill becomes "the novel's ultimate ellipsis".[30] While the traumatic event at the mill remains unspoken, it leaves its mark in a literal puncture through the skin of Marda's hand. Like this wound, the ruin figures the paradox of remembering and forgetting which describes traumatic memory; that is, at once a presence and an absence, the supplement and its void. Marda's wound bears witness to the unspeakable.

This reading of *The Last September*'s traumatized architecture sheds light on Laura's spectral and textual presence in Danielstown;

---

the past. There is a sort of perpetuity about livingness, and it is part of the character of Bowen's Court to be, in sometimes its silent way, very much alive" (*BC* 459).

[26] "The untimeliness is evident in how past, present, and future conspire to converge in the ruin. Having outlived its functional existence, the ruin's persistence in time disproves outright extinction, so compels an unexpected return" (Trigg, *The Aesthetics of Decay*, 131).

[27] Robert Tracy reads Lois and Marda's discovery of the Irish rebel as an encounter with the undead ("Undead, Unburied: Anglo-Ireland and the Predatory Past", *LIT*, X/1 [July 1999], 26-27). See also Julian Moynahan, *Anglo-Irish: The Literary Imagination in a Hyphenated Culture*, Princeton, NJ: Princeton University Press, 1995, 244; Ellmann, *The Shadow Across the Page*, 65.

[28] Trigg, "The Place of Trauma", 99.

[29] *Ibid.*, 95.

[30] Corcoran, "Discovery of a Lack", 327.

she is one of those "indefinite ghosts of the past" Bowen has described, who "add something" to those ancestral homes of the Anglo-Irish.[31] Like the supplement, the ghost is maddeningly "neither presence nor absence". The textual traces Laura has left engraved upon the walls and windows of the house function, like the ruin, as sites of memory and of non-memory. While these traces act as marks of decay upon the Big House, they simultaneously refuse the destruction of their author's memorialization, so that Danielstown comes to act as a tomb for Laura's remains, and moreover, to figure a conflation of the dead woman with the house. If the sign (and here, the signature) does indeed function as supplement for "the thing itself" through that "power of substitution that permits us to absent ourselves and act by proxy", then Laura's textual traces figure the supplement for her absence.[32] Indeed, for Hugo she *is* text: she is, for him, like "some rediscovered diary of a forgotten year" (*LS* 176). Through the novel's repeated acts of reading these traces, Laura is resurrected; she is immortalized in text.

If Laura is supplemented by her textual remains, Danielstown's box-room is her crypt. Thus, in the passage which forms the epigraph to this chapter, Lois chooses that site for a "melanchol[ic]" hiding place (*ibid.*, 192). However, it is not her mother's sign or supplement which Lois seeks, but rather, "the thing itself": her dead mother. The box-room is "too damp for the storage of trunks that were not finished with", and is permeated by a "mustiness [coming] from her mother's old vaulted trunks", and is therefore a site of decay or ruin in the Big House, a "no-place" (when hiding here, Lois is "not anywhere"), a spatio-temporal site of non-memory (*ibid.*, 192).[33] That cleft in Danielstown means that this Big House approaches the traumatized architecture of the mill and mimics the structure of the traumatized psyche, as the box-room forms the site of absence and presence, of memory and non-memory, in the house. Thus, for Lois to "[look and strain] after feeling", but to "[feel] nothing", does not describe an

[31] Elizabeth Bowen, "The Big House" (1940), in *The Mulberry Tree*, 28.

[32] Derrida, "That Dangerous Supplement", 87.

[33] Laura's writing on the box-room wall might also be seen to represent the house's decay (and, indeed, the fall of the Anglo-Irish Ascendancy) in terms of the connotations of "writing on the wall" – supernatural writing which, in the Book of Daniel, predicts the demise of the Babylonian empire.

absence of feeling towards her mother, but rather, suggests that in the box-room she "feels" the "nothingness", the absence of her mother, and moreover, that behind the supplement of the textual and architectural trace, there is the void that represents her mother, "the thing itself".

Furthermore, Lois herself comes to figure a trace or supplement of Laura, "the image of Laura", as she is described throughout the novel (*ibid.*, 4, 17, 84, 87-88, 115); indeed, for Bennett and Royle, "Lois is recognized, known, because she is the image of her mother, a simulacrum or phantom of the dead, a fiction, 'like a novel'".[34] To recognize the girl's spatial negations – she is repeatedly stated to be "nowhere" (*LS* 45, 124, 285) – is then also to recognize the void of Laura for whom her daughter is the sign. But Lois is not only the supplement for her mother; the girl may also be seen as the literal sign of her father, whose absence from the narrative is so profound it is not even remarked upon. All that remains of the elusive Mr Farquar is the patronym borne only by Lois (his wife, Laura, is never referred to by her married name). Lois' own sign, a sign which marks her out as not of this house, not a Naylor, is haunted by a void: the absence of her father. The absence of the girl's parents, then, inflects the way in which Lois "and these home surroundings still penetrated each other mutually in the discovery of a lack" (*ibid.*, 244).

The Last September also works as a supplement for another void: Gerald. Gerald, always already dead, is throughout the novel characterized by a strange non-existence, an inability to be traced (*ibid.*, 80), so that, for example, "his steps on the grass [die] out quickly" (*ibid.*, 122). For Lois to suddenly see "him as though he were dead, as though she had lost him, with the pang of an evocation" (*ibid.*, 70), is to collapse the supplement's charade; swiftly, she revitalizes him in her letter to Viola. Gerald, recognize Bennett and Royle, "cannot be figured, he can only be seen, in fact, dead. Gerald can only be evoked, called from the dead: Gerald can only be described or perceived as if, or if, he was dead."[35] Like those "dead young [men]" in the photographs which fill Mrs Fogarty's drawing-room, whose "candid eyes" one cannot avoid, Gerald is haunted by the spectre of his futurelessness, a death that has always already taken

---

[34] Bennett and Royle, *Elizabeth Bowen and the Dissolution of the Novel*, 17.
[35] *Ibid.*, 21.

place (*LS* 102). "You know I'd die for you", he tells Lois (*ibid.*, 128), but that "you" also addresses the reader in a self-conscious awareness of the novel's inevitable conclusion: Gerald (like Danielstown) must be executed, sacrificed in and for the narrative, even as his own writing "run[s] for [its] life" (*ibid.*, 238).

A conflict has arisen in this chapter's consideration of trauma in spatial terms; that is, in the tension between architectural trauma, the ruin, as a "non-memory", and the monumentalization or immortalization of an event in a structure. Indeed, even though Klaus Lubbers, for example, argues that the Big House in the Big House novel shows "continuity" simply by being, "whether still intact or crumbling", "still there", the voids of that very decay testify to the structure's spatial and temporal uncertainty.[36] That conflict between erasure and immortality, between de(con)struction and preservation, necessarily complicates an understanding of memorialization and trauma in this novel. At its conclusion, then, the narrative opens up a temporal cleft:

> For in February, before those leaves had visibly budded, the death – the execution, rather – of the three houses, Danielstown, Castle Trent, Mount Isabel, occurred in the same night. A fearful scarlet ate up the hard spring darkness; indeed, it seemed that an extra day, unreckoned, had come to abortive birth that these things might happen .... At Danielstown, half way up the avenue under the beeches, the thin iron gate twanged (missed its latch, remained swinging aghast) as the last unlit car slid out with the executioners bland from accomplished duty .... Then the first wave of a silence that was to be ultimate flowed back confidently to the steps ....
>
> Sir Richard and Lady Naylor, not saying anything, did not look at each other, for in the light from the sky they saw too distinctly. (*LS* 303)

That "unreckoned" "extra day" is the "accident of day, of action" of which Laurence's "spectral plot" could not conceive (*ibid.*, 153). This extra day figures a temporal wound in which the novel's trauma occurs: the "execution" of the house. Aflame, the house eats up or

[36] Klaus Lubbers, "Continuity and Change in Irish Fiction: The Case of the Big-House Novel", in *Ancestral Voices: The Big House in Anglo-Irish Literature*, ed. Otto Rauchbauer, Hildesheim: Georg Olms Verlag, 1992, 27.

incorporates the darkness that had earlier threatened it; it swallows, and is swallowed up by, the darkness to which it has been condemned. The novel thus concludes in a climactic and permanent suspension of the traumatic executions of both Danielstown and Gerald, events which Lois does not want to "[get] past", or mourn, but rather maintain (*ibid.*, 299). Indeed, the novel itself does not "get past" these deaths, for its conclusion remains on the house's threshold and in the "aghast" horror of the perpetually swinging gate, as well as in that "wave of a silence" – a "wave" that has been crashing since the announcement of Gerald's murder (*ibid.*, 292). Foreshadowing the conclusion of *Eva Trout*, Danielstown, like Eva, is suspended or stilled in the final trauma, the moment of death. Nothing survives beyond this liminal moment.

CHAPTER 3

REMAINS: *THE HOUSE IN PARIS* AND *FRIENDS AND RELATIONS*

> Everything we read: remains.[1]

> Going into the morning-room, Karen found the pad back on the bureau, where it lived. But it was blank: the message had been torn off – and torn off unprecisely, leaving an edge jagged. The blank pad was scored with curves where writing had dug through; the sheets were thin, her mother's pencil emphatic. Karen stared at it; then, bringing the pad nearer to the light, she took the pencil and traced her mother's dinted writing. What she read was: Karen. 6-30 Saturday. Evelyn Derrick rang you up to talk plans for next week-end. She says will you ring her up on Monday when you are home, before she leaves London?[2]

In *After Derrida*, Nicholas Royle asserts that "All of Derrida's work can be read as an attempt to respond to [the] question of 'remains' – especially, but not only, to the question of 'remains as a written thing'".[3] Cixous also takes up this connection between texts and remains in *Stigmata*, when she makes the provocative statement which forms the epigraph to this chapter: "Everything we read: remains." I want to address this "question of 'remains'" in Bowen's novels *Friends and Relations* and *The House in Paris* as part of an interrogation of the ethics of survival, of reading the trauma narrative, that which remains.

---

[1] Hélène Cixous, "Without End, No, State of Drawingness, No, Rather: The Executioner's Taking Off" (1991), trans. Catherine A.F. MacGillivray, in *Stigmata: Escaping Texts*, 26.

[2] Elizabeth Bowen, *The House in Paris* (1935), Harmondsworth: Penguin, 1976, 171. Hereafter cited parenthetically as *HP*.

[3] Nicholas Royle, *After Derrida*, Manchester: Manchester University Press, 1995, 61.

Friends and Relations and *The House in Paris* explore trauma as narrative traces, or textual ruins – the former novel is haunted by the remains of an alternative narrative plot that threatens to disrupt the present, while the latter incurs disruption as a result of illicitly reading textual remains – but in contrast to the more traditional understanding of trauma and textuality which locates importance in the act of writing and the narrativization of trauma, *The House in Paris* and *Friends and Relations* re-centre ethical responsibility, placing it in the hands of the reader. I agree with Bennett and Royle when they assert that *The House in Paris* is "a traumaturgy, both a work and a theory of wounds", and in this chapter I explore the ways in which that analysis can help us to extend our understanding of trauma theory itself.[4]

Taking up J. Hillis Miller's assertion that the ethical moment "in the act of reading ... is a response to something, responsible for it, responsive to it, respectful of it", I suggest that as part of a Modernist struggle to recognize and represent the cultural and individual traumas of the early twentieth century (and not to live "like a family in a pre-war novel" [*HP* 70]), Bowen's novels explore the ethics of responding to that which survives: the ethics of reading remains.[5] Since, in Royle's terms, "the challenge of Derrida's work as a whole comprises the difficulty of thinking remains *other than on the basis of what was once present*", Derrida's writing can help us to understand Bowen's work in the context of trauma theory and how it might offer a new ethical standpoint on the representation of trauma in narrative. In fact, Derrida challenges the convention of time and consequence when he makes clear that

> The trace, for example, is not the remains of something that was once present and might be rendered present once again: rather it is that which prevents any present, any experience of presence, from being completely itself, from ever coinciding with itself. In the final analysis, then, remains are always and only the remains of remains, just as there are always and only traces of traces.[6]

---

[4] Bennett and Royle, *Elizabeth Bowen and the Dissolution of the Novel*, 43.
[5] J. Hillis Miller, *The Ethics of Reading: Kant, De Man, Eliot, Trollope, James, and Benjamin*, New York: Columbia University Press, 1987, 4.
[6] Royle, *After Derrida*, 61 (original emphasis).

Importantly, this means for both Derrida and Bowen that rather than constituting a negative fragment, in a project of ethical reading remains can come to figure "affirmation itself".[7] The hauntedness of *The House in Paris* and *Friends and Relations* is thus a means to complicate the ways in which we think about secrecy, spectrality, and literature by asking, after trauma, what remains of narrative? How might we who remain, read, after?

Traumatic clairvoyance

The House in Paris adopts a tripartite structure: "The Present", "The Past", "The Present". As in Bowen's later novel, *The Little Girls*, this structure encrypts the past in the present so that the structural analepsis mimics the way in which trauma disrupts the linear progression of time. The "present" sections of the novel span a single day in Paris; Henrietta Arbuthnot, an eleven-year-old girl crossing Paris alone, must spend the day in the care of Naomi Fisher, a friend of her grandmother, while she waits for her evening train. Another child, Leopold, is also present; Leopold was adopted at birth, and will today meet his mother, Karen Forrestier (née Michaelis), for the first time. While the monstrous Mme Fisher, whose house in Paris this is, lies ill overhead, "septic" (*HP* 31) with a past that seeps through the house and its narrative, the two children, left alone, curiously and painfully discuss the secrets of which Naomi has warned them not to speak: "There is no end to the violations committed by children on children, quietly talking alone. Henrietta dreaded what [Leopold] might say next" (*ibid.*, 208). For Henrietta, these "violations" are concerned with the terrifying expectation of reliving the traumatic past – he taunts her with the potential horror of "Helpless" remembering (*ibid.*, 31). Yet when his torture reaches its climax – "You see, you and I are just opposites. I *don't* remember my mother, but *shall* see her again" – the "effect" upon Henrietta is "odd": the girl "seemed to become unconscious of Leopold" (*ibid.*, 32; original emphasis). Henrietta appears to forget her companion, and to push the threat of dredging up the past into her "unconscious". When Karen does not arrive, Leopold, too, must relive the trauma of his infant abandonment. Although he initially mimics Henrietta's response to such provocation, "disengaging himself from [Naomi] and from

---

[7] *Ibid.*, 62.

everyone", his acknowledgement that "my mother is not here" "echoe[s]" and reverberates, returning and repeating back to him the traumatic event of his survival (*ibid.*, 191).

All of this occurs in "The Present". The central section of the novel, "The Past", is narrated from the perspective of Karen, who feels stifled by the restrictions of her upper-middle-class life and longs to revolt against the desires of her mother, and against Ray, Karen's fiancé, for "To be with Ray will be like being with mother" (*ibid.*, 153). Years before, Karen had lived for a year in the house in Paris, then a boarding-house run by Mme Fisher and Naomi for mothers to send "dependable daughters" for whom they wished "freedom inside the bounds of propriety" (*ibid.*, 102). Here Karen had met a young friend of Mme Fisher, Max Ebhart, a man who at once angers and fascinates her (*ibid.*, 99). Naomi's announcement that she is engaged to Max revives Karen's earlier passion for the young man; their illicit affair – brief, but just long enough to conceive Leopold – "is like an epilogue to a book" (*ibid.*, 109). This section of the novel ends after Max's dramatic suicide in the very salon in which Henrietta and Leopold now play, and Karen's subsequent decision to break off her engagement and to travel abroad until after the birth of her child.

Yet, I want to argue that we read this section of the novel as a supposition of Leopold's, narrated by his idea of "the mother who did not come", and who therefore "remained his creature" (*ibid.*, 67): "In the course of that meeting that never happened, that meeting whose scene remained inside Leopold, [Karen] would have told what she had done without looking for motives .... This is, in effect, what she would have had to say." What Karen says, the narrative that forms "The Past" is what Leopold supplies her with, what he imagines "she would have had to say" if she had come to visit as he had expected, if she had spoken to him "as he had thought she would" (*ibid.*, 68). Leopold's story becomes a kind of survivor narrative as the child reads himself as remains. The child does not, cannot know the events that "made me be" (*ibid.*, 67); indeed, he "swelled with content at his own ignorance of the past" (*ibid.*, 193). But the meeting of Leopold and Karen is a narrative of a never-arriving future for which we are always waiting, even at the novel's conclusion; the novel simply leaves us, in transit, on a station platform.

The House in Paris frustrates the narrative of Leopold's expectation of remembrance, formed by the remains of a "meeting whose scene remained inside" him, in order to reject an understanding of healing through resolution. The ethics of survival cannot solely depend on a cohesion which, as this case testifies, may never happen. Rather, the model of trauma Bowen proposes is one which reads remains as irreconcilable with that which was "once present," and indeed, that such a reading would not, in any case, be the point. An ethical reading of trauma, this chapter argues, recognizes remains as survival, as affirmation, and thus resituates the conventional traumatic affect.

Aftermath

The House in Paris is an aftermath. All we read are remains. Each of the many ellipses, which occur more frequently than in Bowen's other novels, figures another "crack across the crust of life" (*ibid.*, 127), another "crack [in] the tomb" (*ibid.*, 203), another shattered alabaster lid that traces the remains of a traumatic history (*ibid.*, 212). In this way, *The House in Paris* is constructed from the remains of the traumatic past: the narrative itself is the "young tree inside a tomb" which "discover[s] the power to crack the tomb and grow up to any height" (*ibid.*, 203). All of this means that the second section of the novel, "The Past", in which the story of the illicit love affair between Karen and Max Ebhart is played out, is itself a fictional construct arising from the "clairvoyant" act of Leopold Grant Moody, the product – the remains – of this affair. Just as he "thought-read[s]" from the empty envelope, Leopold reads into and writes over the silences that surround his existence (*ibid.*, 59). The novel's central section, "The Past", similarly works as supplement to the present, growing through those cracks in the tomb, the hanging pause after Naomi's momentous announcement: "Your mother is not coming; she cannot come" (*ibid.*, 66, 191). This sentence appears twice in the novel: at the conclusion of the first section entitled "The Present", and to introduce the resumption of the present in the third section. By framing "The Past" with a repetition of the same sentence, the text works to hide the events of the second section; no time has passed in the present while we have read "The Past". By returning the reader to precisely the point at which narration of "The Present" was left, the novel refuses that narrative of "The Past". As no time has passed, no narrative could have happened, this repetition asserts. *The House in Paris* remains tight-lipped: we cannot ethically read the past from its remains in the present.

Cixous' reading of Derrida's *Circumfessions* and its scattered "remains" is uncannily reminiscent of (perhaps even ghosted by) *The House in Paris*; it puts Leopold in mind and moreover, puts in mind "the questions he had kept waiting so long for [Karen]", those questions which she never arrives to answer: "Why am I? What made me be?" (*ibid.*, 67) The mother "at the last moment, when he asked her 'who am I?' did not answer him", notes Cixous of Derrida's text; "she never was able to answer the question what am I":

> We need the mother's acknowledgement, she's the one we ask for the words ..., the word that glues the pieces back together again. When she doesn't answer for me, I am broken. But how should she answer for a me? I am lodged in incapacity and there I remain me on one hand my name on the other, the name calls me and who am I to answer? Here I remain, here I am a remains ....
>
> She remains to him, in leaving, after her departure, like those questions without response that come back to haunt us.[8]

Part of what is so interesting about *The House in Paris* is that Karen may be said to play out (or to be haunted by) the logic of the mother as articulated by Cixous and Derrida. How should the mother answer for the child, how should Karen answer for Leopold's existence, how should she answer for what remains of the past? The "indecipherable, evasive" mother for Derrida and in this novel, for Leopold, maintains her narrative silence: she "keeps her secret", she fails to speak for herself and, therefore, for her child.[9] It is precisely because she remains silent that Leopold must imagine her testimony to his "broken" identity and construct a spectral interruption to the present.

The central section of the novel seems to seek to "answer for a me", for although it narrates the past, this portion of the text is fixated on Leopold as its sole issue. Leopold's imagination of Karen's testimony is prefaced by a statement of memory untainted, of the past

---

[8] Hélène Cixous, *Portrait of Jacques Derrida as a Young Jewish Saint*, trans. Beverley Bie Brahic, New York: Columbia University Press, 2004, 51-52.

[9] *Ibid.*, 52.

cinematically replayed with careful unawareness of the future, "the whole being": "You suppose the spools of negatives that are memory (from moments when the whole being was, unknown, exposed), developed without being cut for a false reason: entire letters, dialogues which, once spoken, remain spoken for ever being unwound from the dark, word by word" (*HP* 68). However, the recurring sense of anticipation and awareness of the future in this section betrays Leopold's fictional retrospection: it is pregnant with the thought of the future, of him. Endlessly, the novel's many clocks "march ticking on through the dark" (*ibid.*, 87), moving ever forward to the inevitable child, mimicking the tick-tock of Karen's perpetual thought, "What next? What next?" (*ibid.*, 69). The atmosphere of Aunt Violet and Uncle Bill's home, where "The Past" begins, is great with the anticipation of death – "what was going to happen stood at the door" (*ibid.*, 86). Karen's inescapable future is foreshadowed when she reads this prospect "as though those two were a couple expecting their first child" (*ibid.*, 82). Immediately, this fictional remembering is directed towards its intertwined conclusions of birth (Leopold) and death (Max).

Karen's expectations for the first year of her marriage also project the seeming paradox of the anticipation of memory; she looks to a now foreign future made familiar – to a strange child, to unknown "times of day in the future house, making tomorrow fatten thin today" (*ibid.*, 124). In the same way that Leopold imagines the moment of his mother's arrival as an event soon to be part of memory – "From that door opening, I shall remember on .... I shall see what I cannot imagine now" – so too Karen's narrative is concerned with the making of memory, with what will in future remain of the past (*ibid.*, 40). This is the temporal reflexivity to which Karen refers when she states that "something in Ireland bends one back on oneself" (*ibid.*, 89). To "bend back", in *The House in Paris*, is to consider the present from the perspective of the future, a desire to "give the future something to talk about" (*ibid.*, 144).[10] And, if it is true, as Bowen states in "The

[10] The link between this statement and Bowen's essay, "The Bend Back", is adequately explored in extant criticism. See, for example, Timothy Dow Adams, "'Bend Sinister': Duration in Elizabeth Bowen's *The House in Paris*", *International Fiction Review*, 7 (1980), 51, and Lee's *Elizabeth Bowen*, which includes a chapter entitled "The Bend Back".

Bend Back" (1950), that "It is not the past but the idea of the past which draws us", it might be seen that the present, in this novel, only holds fascination in terms of an abstracted becoming-past, a becoming-memory.[11]

Leopold's desire to foresee the future of his meeting with Karen – to know not only "what made me be", but what will make him be – and his demand that Henrietta tell his fortune using a pack of cards, is also a longing to know the past. It is for this reason, perhaps, that Henrietta's reading of the future confuses narrative time and real time, for her prediction of death when Leopold turns up the ten of spades is for the novel's future, rather than Leopold's (*HP* 64). Henrietta's fortune-telling at once summons Max's suicide in the historical past and foresees it in the future of the novel's "The Past". But the boy wishes not so much to know the future, but rather, he says, to "[make] things happen", to make memory. His destruction of Henrietta's occult circle of cards when she fails to "make anything come" might thus be read as an attempt to erase or to hide the beginning of a memory formation with which he is dissatisfied (*ibid.*, 65). But he is too late, the cards are dealt; they call forth the predicted future through the messenger Miss Fisher, who insists that "Something unforeseen must have happened" (*ibid.*, 193), even while her "eyes streamed as she rode at him like the figurehead of a ship" (*ibid.*, 66) – the very "gilt ship" which adorns the backs of Henrietta's "foreseeing" cards (*ibid.*, 65).

For Bennett and Royle, this clairvoyant concern for an unavoidable future is figured by the repetitions of the word "dread" in the novel; dread, they point out, "suggests a fear of future events, a fear grounded in the present ... the subject of dread is caught up in – already dreading, and therefore already experiencing – the event which is dreaded".[12] Dread, then, might be seen to engage a temporal reversal of traumatic memory, the unbidden re-experiencing of the past, in what we might call a traumatic clairvoyance, an unbidden "already experiencing" of the future. Indeed, it is in Henrietta's clairvoyant act that the novel might be seen to be "already experiencing" its own traumatic future – Max's suicide and Leopold's hidden identity. Max's fate is foreseen, or already experienced in the

---

[11] Elizabeth Bowen, "The Bend Back" (1950), in *The Mulberry Tree*, 58.

[12] Bennett and Royle, *Elizabeth Bowen and the Dissolution of the Novel*, 61.

text, first when Henrietta remembers "how much blood had been shed in Paris" (*HP* 22), and then at least twice by Max himself who, when Naomi accidentally pricks herself with a needle, "wished the blood were on my own finger" (*ibid.*, 162), and admits to Karen that "When I cut myself even slightly, I bleed like a pig, profusely" (*ibid.*, 139). This anticipation of bloodshed works against Naomi's belief that Max "had foreseen nothing", and against Mme Fisher's insistence that "no trace led us" to Max's remains (*ibid.*, 183, 185).

The House in Paris does not only foresee its own conclusion: to read *The House in Paris* is to be "already experiencing" the traumatic future of Bowen's later writing. This novel twice anticipates the violent conclusion to *Eva Trout*: when Karen imagines "whipping a pistol out of her kid bag and firing" (*ibid.*, 125), and when Ray recognizes in Leopold that "A child knows what is fatal" (*ibid.*, 220). "The child at the back of the gun accident", Ray asks, "is he always so ignorant? I simply point this thing, it goes off" (*ibid.*, 220). Aunt Violet's death, too, is felt by Karen and by the reader to greater effect prior to this traumatic event – "She died before this, thought Karen" (*ibid.*, 128). Karen's mother and father, however, had not anticipated this trauma: "Everyone blamed Uncle Bill for letting Aunt Violet's death come as such a shock; Karen did not even ask herself why *she* had said nothing" (*ibid.*, 131). She does not ask herself why she had said "nothing" – an act which prefigures her later deceptions – indeed, more precisely, why Karen had said of her aunt, "*She* said nothing", when questioned by Mrs Michaelis (emphasis added). In protecting her mother from dread, from a traumatic "already experiencing" of the future, Karen also prevents her mother from experiencing in the present, as "the shock" of this sudden knowledge means that she does not "feel anything else yet" (*ibid.*, 127). Later, it is suggested that the death of Mrs Michaelis was hastened by "the shock of her sister's death" (and, circumspectly, by the shock of her daughter's pre-marital pregnancy) – in short, she is shocked to death by Karen's lies (*ibid.*, 219).

Bowen critiques the temporal instability offered up by traumatic clairvoyance in the sense that one cannot ever truly know the past, just as one cannot know the future. She therefore troubles our understanding of trauma as seeing or knowing too late (in Caruth's terms) precisely by pointing out the impossibility of this hermeneutic model.

Thought (re)reading

A kind of textual haunting or anticipation also inflects Leopold's "spectral reading" of his mother's thoughts, not only in relation to the central section of the narrative, but also when he discovers in Naomi's handbag an empty envelope which had contained a letter from his mother. Leopold attempts a kind of psychic dictation of the absent note:

> Getting up and pushing back the chairs, he began to pace the salon, with his eyes shut, pressing her empty envelope to his forehead as he had once seen a thought-reader do. Then he began to read slowly aloud, as though the words one by one passed under his eyelids: "Dear Miss Fisher," he said. (*Ibid.*, 45)

Yet Leopold is not reading his mother's thoughts, but rather his own. Thus, he again projects his own desires onto those of his mother, for he believes that "She's the same as me; she would see why I do things" (*ibid.*, 59). His insistence upon psychological symbiosis with a woman he has not met "since he can remember" gives him, he thinks, moral permission to not only touch her letters, but to appropriate her voice, to write this letter and later, to write the past, in her name (*ibid.*, 20).[13] Leopold thus reads the absence or secret of the missing letter, the missing mother, from what remains: himself. That is, like a detective, Leopold hunts for textual clues to his mother's past, delving into Henrietta's suitcase and into Miss Fisher's handbag "with the immediate thought that inside there might be letters about him" (*HP* 39). Yet Leopold is not only the detective, but also already the evidence of the crime, the fingerprint at the scene, the "mark … on the grass" which, in the novel, comes to signify Max and Karen's illicit

---

[13] Henrietta informs Leopold of this moral code when she finds him "thought-reading" the letter: "It's dishonourable to *touch* other people's letters" (*HP* 59). "To Henrietta", note Bennett and Royle, "Leopold's 'reading' transgresses the conventions both of sanity … and of a kind of insane decorum" (*Elizabeth Bowen and the Dissolution of the Novel*, 48). Moreover, in *Friends and Relations*, Edward is similarly horrified when Janet asks to read a letter not written to her: "'No, I couldn't,' said Edward, appalled. 'That would be absolutely impossible!'" (*FR* 88).

touch and the commencement of their romantic affair (*ibid.*, 153). Leopold is what remains of Karen's lie, and he seeks to expose her as the perpetrator of his traumatic survival.

Karen's lies and silences, her unexplained absences, continue in the present. As I have already noted, Leopold (and the reader) must reread his mother's absence: twice, Naomi's news is reported. Yet this traumatic repetition is not over:

> "Because my mother is not here."
>
> Leopold, having said this in an experimentary voice, stopped to hear it echoed, looking, meanwhile, self-compellingly at and through Henrietta, as though "*My mother is not here*," were written all over her – face, dress, hair – and he were forcing himself to read it again and again and again. (*Ibid.*, 195; original emphasis)

Aurally and textually, Karen's absence is repeated, echoed, reread. To live through trauma once "is enough", Karen admits to Naomi; nevertheless, she forces her child to endure recurring abandonment (*ibid.*, 186). Over and over she is not coming, she does not come; over and over Leopold anticipates, (re)experiences the trauma of yet another of Karen's betrayals, rereading Mme Fisher's unauthorized assertion, "That she must not love you was written on her heart" (*ibid.*, 207). Leopold exhibits a Freudian "compulsion to repeat" (or to reread) the traumatic event, the trauma of abandonment, as he "self-compellingly … forc[es] himself to read it again and again and again". In this way, rereading is proposed as analogous to the traumatic repetitions of the psyche, the unconscious drive to revisit and to work through the memory of trauma.[14]

It is the simultaneous compulsion to repeat and to reread the past, and yet to refuse its irruption into the present, with which Karen appears to struggle. It is her desire to see Leopold again which precipitates the novel's action, but this reunion does not take place within the narrative, and in the novel's final moments, Ray refuses to respond to the child's hopeful question, "Will my mother come tonight?" (*HP* 239). Karen "dreads the past", Leopold and Mme

[14] Freud describes the "compulsion to repeat" earlier traumas, in dream, in memory, or in reality, in *Beyond the Pleasure Principle* (1920), and argues that this arises, in part, from the need to mourn, or to work through the trauma (in *The Essentials of Psycho-Analysis*, 240-41).

Fisher recognize repeatedly (*ibid*., 207, 215, 220). But this is a dread specifically concerned with a fear of traumatic return, a dread not of the past, but of "already experiencing" the past again, of "already experiencing" a future act of remembering. Just as Leopold taunts Henrietta with the threat of remembering the trauma of her mother's death, the dread of remembering Leopold himself tortures helpless Karen. From the moment Karen expects Leopold, she denies the remains of her affair while her uncertain tone expects the horror of remembering: "No, there is nothing *to* regret. I mean, there is nothing left now, is there, nothing?" (*ibid*., 164). For Karen and for Leopold, the novel is a narrative of expectation, but for her, it is also a narrative of its denial. Her wish, in the "unspoken dialogue" between her and her husband, "to be back where we started", is to return to a time prior to the traumatic past, the remains of which she would in future dread (*ibid*., 216):

> SHE: ... I don't remember. I never remember. It's time you stopped .... I want to be alone with you. Stop remembering.
> HE: It is you who remember.
> SHE: All I want is for us to be alone.
> HE: We are not alone: there is Leopold .... we are never alone, while you're dreading him. It is you who remember. If he were here with us, he'd be simply a child, either in or out of the room. While he is a dread of yours, he is everywhere ....
> SHE: Stop feeding on my experience. (*Ibid*., 216-17)

Karen's refusal to acknowledge the past, to consign memory as she had consigned Leopold, also figures the Freudian compulsion to repeat, a cycle she imposes upon Leopold when she repeats her abandonment of him, and a cycle Ray seeks to work through by arranging their reunion. Yet Karen accuses Ray of appropriating her trauma, of "feeding on my experience". Parasitic, Ray, like Leopold, illicitly reads her past. The two of them feed on her remains, on the "violets she had pinned on for Leopold pressed dead between her breast and the bed", on her "deadly [quiet]" voice (*ibid*., 215), and on the "dead child" (*ibid*., 205) whose birth precipitated Karen's decision to have Leopold adopted. The compulsion of Karen and Ray to repeat this "circular" dialogue suggests that this cycle of remembering "has no end". If this dialogue resurfaces "when you least expect" – when you least dread – Karen must always be on her guard against Ray's remembering (*ibid*., 218). But in doing so, as Ray points out, Karen herself remembers. To dread and to cease to dread the past thus presents a double-bind in this novel, for both permit trauma to resurface.

Textual traces

It is, then, the traumatic remains of Karen's lies, Karen's secrets, which structure the novel. She, like her son, practises illegal reading activity; feeling like "a thief in her own house", in a kind of act of "thought-reading" which foreshadows and, in the temporal multiplicity of this novel, echoes Leopold's, Karen reads the remains of her mother's lie in order to read her own secret (*ibid*., 170). In what I think is one of the most important moments in the novel, given as the second epigraph to this chapter, Karen returns from a secret weekend with Max. Her mother asks with whom she had stayed; Karen, lying, tells her that she had stayed with a friend, Evelyn, but after her mother has gone to bed, discovers the reason for her unexplained behaviour. Gradually, Karen reads the remains of her own lie between the lines of her mother's reminder, a note which insists on reminding her, on putting in Karen's mind, and in her hand, her own secret. (Mme Fisher's request that Mrs Michaelis tell Karen "that she is in my mind often", is a similarly threatening "reminder" [*ibid*., 130].) In the ghost of her mother's lie, Karen reads the textual remains of her own secret. Everything we read: remains.

Mrs Michaelis' note might then be seen to parallel Leopold's conception for both are acts which produce traces and which give away the secret affair. Mrs Michaelis' writing performs an act which her upbringing does not permit her; that is, it allows her to confront her daughter with her lie. Julian Wolfreys comments on Cixous' phrase, "Everything we read: remains", that it "simultaneously keeps its secrets and reveals them, placing them in plain view, in the light of day".[15] And in a similar way, Mrs Michaelis' text not only enacts the secrets which haunt *The House in Paris*, but also the very secrecy of literature, what Derrida describes as "the right to say everything or to say without saying, and thus the right to the secret displayed as

[15] Julian Wolfreys, *Readings: Acts of Close Reading in Literary Theory*, Edinburgh: Edinburgh University Press, 2000, 32.

such".[16] Mrs Michaelis' note, I suggest, is the site of the novel's trauma: the expected remains of Leopold. Note that Leopold and Henrietta spend almost all of the narrative in the room in which Max had committed suicide. Moreover, Max does not leave a suicide note, but does leave his unborn son, and might then be said to haunt the present in the form of his son. These multiple traces mean that Leopold might also be seen to be the site of, and in the site of, another traumatic spectre: his father. Leopold is the textual trace Mrs Michaelis at once leaves and does not leave, just as he is the bruising mark on the grass left and yet not left by Karen and Max's "unexploring, consenting touch", and the ghostly effect of Henrietta's palm print on the table (*HP* 120).

Leopold is the narrative's secret – he is what is simultaneously hidden and revealed as textual remains. In these compounding acts of spectral reading, then, Leopold seeks to shatter the "husk of silence" that surrounds his existence, to trace the remains of his mother's lie and thus to testify to his own survival (*ibid.*, 219). "Here I remain", as Cixous has it, "here I am a remains". Leopold manipulates the narrative in order to memorialize himself, to remove himself from a site of forgetting in which that trace of his birth, and of his birth name, is consigned to secrecy.

> "Her name's Forrestier."
> ...
> "Then why are you Grant Moody?"
> "Because no one knows I'm born." (*Ibid.*, 59)

Leopold seeks to overcome his uncertain figuration as traumatic "remains" by insisting on his presence – that he remains. In these processes of reading remains and in the revelation of secrets, both Karen and Leopold make Leopold known; they read Leopold, an illegitimate inscription, into being, and affirm, rather than negate, his survival.

---

[16] Jacques Derrida, *Paper Machine*, trans. Rachel Bowlby, Stanford, CA: Stanford University Press, 2005, 163. See also my discussion of Bowen's narrative secrets in Chapter 8.

Narrative familiar

To read *Friends and Relations* is also to read remains. In *Bowen's Court*, Bowen asks: "does vacuum fill the life one has not chosen to live?" (*BC* 444) In this part of the chapter, I want to think about the operation of that unlived life in Bowen's often overlooked novel *Friends and Relations*, and to suggest that it is haunted, in a sense, by a familiar, by the remains of an alternative narrative plot that threatens to disrupt the present. In other words, *Friends and Relations* is haunted by another story, a parallel tale invisibly played out through its textual trace. But as in *The House in Paris*, in *Friends and Relations*, Bowen plays with a kind of narratological simulacra as she troubles the task of locating originary trauma. In this novel, to "bend back" is disruptive rather than redemptive.

Bowen's third novel also adopts a tripartite structure; the first section, "Edward and Rodney", opens on the morning of Laurel and Edward's wedding, the "Tilney-Studdart wedding", and on the steady rain which rouses in the "bride's relations", and in the reader, "a sense of doom" (*FR* 7). Nevertheless, the happy couple depart for their honeymoon unscathed, and before their return, Laurel's sister, Janet, has also become engaged, to Rodney Meggatt. Yet "a cruel obstacle" (*ibid.*, 15) appears: Rodney, rather unfortunately, is discovered to be the nephew of Considine Meggatt, the "co-respondent" (*ibid.*, 16) of Edward's mother, Lady Elfrida, in her divorce from Edward's father. A fuss made by Edward leads to the brief breaking of this engagement, but the couple are reconciled, and the section concludes with Janet and Rodney's marriage. The second and third sections, "The Fine Week" and "Wednesday", take place ten years later; three children – Anna and Simon Tilney, and Hermione Meggatt – have been produced, and the families live more or less harmoniously in London (the Tilneys) and at Batts (the Meggatts' country home). However, the presence of Lady Elfrida and Considine at Batts during the time at which Anna and Simon are staying upsets Edward, who arrives, "without warning, furious, in a fly, without a suitcase, to take away his children who were being corrupted" (*ibid.*, 91). In the wake of this scandal, on one seemingly endless Wednesday, Edward and Janet impotently attempt to ignite an affair, a "large non-occurrence" (*ibid.*, 144) which Corcoran calls "the novel's partially obscured plot of unrealized adultery".[17] Nothing happens, and each returns to their family.

The many clocks of Bowen's fiction are perhaps most remarkable in *Friends and Relations*. Laurel's "cupidy clock", with a "heart on its pendulum" (*FR* 121), literally beats time, while Janet's "loud clocks" invade the quietude of her country house (*ibid.*, 51). However, the clocks of *Friends and Relations* are "imperfectly synchronized, deepening the moment" (*ibid.*, 146). Time, in this novel, seems to proceed on two planes, one the present narrative, the other a "deepen[ed]" narrative in which Edward and Janet marry; the "two clocks" which the latter "allowed … to tick" when Edward attempts to break her engagement to Rodney might be seen to measure these two alternative narrative paths (*ibid.*, 46). Indeed, as he waits for Janet, Edward's mind is itself "no more than a clock where each minute struck like a little hour, with such a reverberation among his senses that the hum of the restaurant was retarded …. This clang of over-charged minutes pointed the irony of those years" (*ibid.*, 113). The time they have together, the stolen time of the relationship that should have been, is marked, in Edward's mind, on its own scale. The present is paused, "retarded", while the "over-charged minutes" not only carry the significance of Edward's wait, but foreshadow the "over-draft" Janet feels she has on time (*ibid.*, 129). Their time is extra, extraneous to the narrative present, borrowed from that other temporal plane, that other narrative which ghosts this novel.

The present in this novel appears as a protracted mistake: it is as if the characters persist in living lives that should not have been lived. The obsession with the possibility of an alternative narrative which so haunts and disrupts the novelistic present can be traced to the illicit affair of Lady Elfrida and Considine. It is the memory or remains of Elfrida and Considine's passion which infects the younger generation with a desire for the same, as Laurel recognizes. Like *The House in Paris*, then, *Friends and Relations* is a novel concerned with the after-effects of adultery, with what remains of a foundational trauma, "the old branching sin like the fatal apple-tree" (*ibid.*, 99). Anna and Hermione, for example, seem to have each been born to the wrong parents: the former "was fair, like Laurel, and would have been a suitable daughter for Rodney" (*ibid.*, 59), while Hermione is "A

[17] Corcoran, *The Enforced Return*, 2.

preposterous child for Janet" (*ibid.*, 53).[18] To read the traces of an alternative genealogy in these girls is to recognize the novel's familiar, to read the narrative that should have been.

Moreover, while the novel's conclusion appears to seek a return to the narrative fork in the road, as it were, and to reconstruct the Studdart family of Laurel and Janet's girlhood, it seems to me possible that this conclusion is, rather, a penetration to the novel's parallel narrative that refuses to acknowledge the survival of descendants in the present. Laurel's regressive behaviour during these final visits to her parents' home forms an undoing of what we know of her experience in the novel: when she returns home it is as if "She has never been away" (*ibid.*, 151):

> Laurel Tilney's coming occasioned far more disturbance ....
>
> Her old room, her white-painted bed should have seemed very narrow. Once or twice Mrs Studdart looked in, very late, to find Laurel curled up on her side, staring at the shell-shadow the electric light shade always cast on the ceiling .... In the darkness there was a movement, as though Laurel held her arms out, as though she were nine years old. Her mother continued: "Does Anna stare at the light?"
>
> "Anna?"
>
> Yes, her coming again and again occasioned disturbance; it was like a birth in the house. She affected the very clocks; nothing seemed quite in order .... They had married her well, properly, formally, with a marquee; but they had not, somehow, married her *off*. She remained .... In talk, Mrs Studdart again and again felt it proper to pick up Laurel's life, like a piece of unfinished sewing, and hand it back to her. Had she mislaid the pattern? (*Ibid.*, 148-50; original emphasis)

Laurel is like a ghost that cannot be exorcized: "She remained." She repeatedly abandons her life as a Tilney, leaving it "like a piece of unfinished sewing" in order to take up the life it seems she should have had. The temporal "disturbance[s]" her visits bring about, "affect[ing] the very clocks", are "like a birth" – like another life, a life of which the "pattern" had been "mislaid". Most importantly, however, Laurel here forgets her daughter, product of a marriage that should not have been. Anna's existence, part of the trauma of Laurel's

[18] Simon, unlike the two girls, "could be left out of any discussion, he was a pure Studdart with a square head like his grandfather's" (*FR* 58).

mislived life, is forgotten; or rather, Laurel is unable to remember Anna because she exists only on the narrative plane of *Friends and Relations*, while Laurel here inhabits the spectral plane of her unlived life.[19] It is as if Laurel's identity has suffered a temporal split, embodying those "imperfectly synchronized" clocks that echo throughout her home: while one Laurel drove away to begin her married life, "a frightful mistake" (*ibid.*, 123), and "never once looked round" (*ibid.*, 150), another Laurel spectrally "remained" at Corunna Lodge (*ibid.*, 110-11). Laurel does not desire to return within the context of her present life; rather, she wishes to reject "her now so ghostly present" for life, for reality as it should have been. In this way, the two planes of the novel are formed – the narrative and its familiar, the life of order and the "patch of ghostly new carpet" that threatens to disturb it (*ibid.*, 121).

The evening on which Edward and Janet share their illicit rendezvous represents one of the temporal folds of traumatic recognition which bring together these two planes of the novel. However, it is Laurel and, moreover, Anna, helplessly awaiting Edward's return, who recognize this transgression not only of the Tilney's marriage, but of time itself:

> At half-past four – by the stroke of three clocks imperfectly synchronized, so that the moment was in itself protracted, deformed – Laurel ceased to expect him .... After this no more clocks struck, something had died down somewhere or been arrested. She rang up the exchange to hear a voice, to be told the time. This verified the solidity of the hour ....
>
> Anna suddenly asked: "You are speaking the truth, aren't you?" Drawing sharply away, scarlet, she said: "*Has he been arrested*?" (*Ibid.*, 133-34; original emphasis)

Here, the narrative and its familiar overlap; indeed, they might almost be seen to interrupt one another. Such overlaps make us privy to the novel's disjointed time, and to the traumatic realization of transgressions which mutate time, make it "protracted, deformed", and beyond the scope of a single linear plane.

---

[19] The way in which Laurel holds her arms out to her mother also recalls Hermione's physical yearning for Janet: "Hermione's face came up in the dark, her arms, her whole body" (*FR* 60).

In seeking a romantic meeting with Janet, and thus playing out a part of the novel's spectral plot (that is, Janet and Edward's marriage), Edward disorders and corrupts the temporality of *Friends and Relations*. While Laurel suspects that her husband's absence might be explained by such disjuncture, it is Anna who voices the criminality of Edward's behaviour: "*Has he been arrested*?" Indeed, the question of his arrest is not only in relation to the law, but also to time. It is midnight when Edward and Janet part, a liminal moment of arrest, neither Tuesday nor Wednesday (*ibid*., 128). Having transgressed the temporal (and moral) boundaries of the life he chose when he married Laurel, Edward is conceived of as arrested: "There was, all at once, nowhere for Edward to go; he felt too old for his world; he had graduated" (*ibid*., 124). Criminal, "disorderly", he no longer adheres to the temporal structure of *Friends and Relations*, but has "nowhere … [else] to go". Thus, he remains arrested, stilled between the two narrative planes, between the two sisters. It might be seen that this terrifying arrest is foreshadowed by Hermione's nightmare: "I had a frightful dream; I dreamed I was nowhere" (*ibid*., 104). For Hermione to dream she is "nowhere" is to imagine the alternative life in which she did not exist – traumatic thought of absence for a child. To implore her mother to "go on holding me tight, don't go; I wish we were the same person!" (*ibid*., 104) is, then, not only a desire for pre-Oedipal symbiosis, as Elizabeth Cullingford posits, but a desire to overcome the possibility of her mother's solitary slippage into an alternative life, a threatening spectre that invades even the child's psyche.[20]

This sense of a temporal and narrative multiplicity is also made manifest through the way in which characters are thought to haunt other spaces; it as if, we, like Lady Elfrida, have "always been seeing something over [Laurel's] shoulder" (*FR* 123). At another of these temporal folds – Janet and Edward's discussion of the fatal letter sent by Theodora Thirdman, which has occasioned his urgent visit – the very room in which they stand is "now empty of Janet and Edward, as though both had turned and gone out by different doors, or had never come in" (*ibid*., 87). As the memory of their early secret passion is raised, their very presence in the present is made impossible. It is as if

[20] Elizabeth Cullingford, "'Something Else': Gendering Onliness in Elizabeth Bowen's Early Fiction", *Modern Fiction Studies*, LIII/2 (Summer 2007), 294.

they "had never come in", never had occasion for this interview, never continued on their mistaken narrative paths. Similarly, Rodney is plagued by anxiety when Janet is away from him: "Her absences, which he would hardly admit as absences, penetrated and racked him. Before death she had ghosts all over the house; she was preceded and followed" (*ibid.*, 52). For Rodney, Janet herself is multiplied, or rather, shadowed, by a disjointed or disordered self. She exists both before and after herself. What frightens Rodney, it seems, is the possibility that Janet might leave their marriage, that she might choose her alternative narrative. He, like Laurel, becomes aware of the spectre of this other temporal plane, and sees this hauntedness in a multiplicity of Janet herself. Similarly, Laurel sees Edward out of time, as someone who should be elsewhere, but who is briefly, illicitly, present, "as though Edward were someone to whom she had already said good-bye, who had left her then slipped back for something forgotten; someone in haste, unwilling to be detained, impossible to accost, so that she must only secretly watch through the crack of a door or over the banisters his ghostly coming and going" (*ibid.*, 125).

In the most eerie of these temporal disjunctions, this "duality" (*ibid.*, 117) is disturbed by a spectral third sister, ghostly intermediary between Laurel and Janet:

> These weeks, a grotesque, not quite impossible figure, had come to interpose between herself and Laurel. A woman, an unborn shameful sister, travestying their two natures, enemy to them both .... Where had the three met, how did the two, innocent, recognize the third? We know *of* her, we do not know her .... Laurel once said: "Do you notice, it's always the same woman whose letters are read in court?" This ever-presence in profile had, for each of the sisters, the Egyptian effective defect: from Janet's side or from Laurel's – could either have seen her, she was so close, or, faced her, she was so dreadful – two eyes were visible, focussed elsewhere with an undeviating intentness. The look directed upon Edward its whole darkness. (*Ibid.*, 116-17)

This "grotesque ... figure", I suggest, is the spectre of Laurel and Janet's other lives, the "unborn" woman each might have been, the witness "in court" to "shameful" narrative and moral transgression: their unborn family, their unborn relation, their dark familiar. A similar spectre is also present to Mrs Studdart, who "had a confidante, an intimate always present, who did not exist. A lady …. In fact, a kind of sublime Mrs Studdart" (*ibid.*, 150). But the description of this figure as "the third" tempts a link with Theodora Thirdman, she who harbours lesbian desires for Janet, and whose meddling letter brings about what might have been the fall of the two houses.

It is Theodora's letter which is read aloud by Janet as evidence for Edward's removal of his children; Theodora's letter which prompts Laurel's realization of the love harboured by Edward and Janet. It is Theodora's letter, then, which brings about the overlap of the novel and its familiar. This third figure is a kind of Medusa whose "dreadful" gaze is "directed upon Edward", if not as a rival for Janet's affection, then as a representation of the novel's hinge, the one whose marital error divides the narrative. Edward's "arrest", then, is a result of the Medusa's deadly stare, as he wavers between the two sisters, between the novel's two narrative planes, and is caught by their unnamed third. All of the Studdart women, then, are shadowed by a familiar, a kind of omniscient friend or relation that I suggest is a figure of the doubled narrative. That is if, as I have argued, the narrative is haunted, then it follows that each character may be split into a present-self, and its shadow, the remains of a self-that-might-have-been. It is this self-that-might-have-been which figures the haunting familiar of the surviving Studdart women, and indeed, of *Friends and Relations* itself.

Torn texts

> Karen suddenly, but with intense calm, took Max's letter to Naomi from her pocket, read the address then tore it across four times …. She glanced once at the water, but scattered the scraps on the wet grass, where they lay like the broken trail of a paper chase. (*HP* 164)

> [Janet] still had the letter; she looked from the letter into the fireplace, but there was nothing but cold, stacked logs. So more or less absently and without ostentation she tore and re-tore the letter across. (*FR* 89)

In both *The House in Paris* and *Friends and Relations*, the textual traces of adultery are destroyed: the letter of confession Max composes to Naomi is torn and scattered by Karen, marking the grass as their transgressive hands had done, while Theodora's meddling revelation to Laurel is shredded by Janet. This repetition of textual destruction appears to suggest that piecing a text back together is not only impossible, but not the point: trauma, insistently, remains, even demands, to be read. In these novels, "everything we read: remains"; everything we read is the remains of those shredded secrets. In this way, *The House in Paris* and *Friends and Relations* appear to anticipate, to think through, and perhaps, to ghost Cixous' and Derrida's question of remains in terms of their engagement with trauma and identity. These novels complicate and extend our understanding of the intersections between trauma, secrecy, and spectrality in narrative, and most importantly, our understanding of reading as an ethical demand in response to survival.

CHAPTER 4

DEATH SLEEP: *THE DEATH OF THE HEART*

> I've heard [*The Death of the Heart*], for instance, called a tragedy of adolescence. I never thought of it that way when I wrote it and I must say I still don't see it in that way now. The one adolescent character in it, the young girl Portia seems to me to be less tragic than the others. She at least, has a hope, and she hasn't atrophied. The book is really a study, it might be presumptuous of me to call it a tragedy of atrophy, not of death so much as of death sleep. And the function of Portia in the story is to be the awake one, in a sense therefore she was a required character. She imparts meaning rather than carries meaning.[1]

> To remember can be at times no more than a cold duty, for we remember only in the limited way that is bearable. We observe small rites, but we defend ourselves against that terrible memory that is stronger than will. We defend ourselves from the rooms, the scenes, the objects that make for hallucination, that make the senses start up and fasten upon a ghost. We desert those who desert us; we cannot afford to suffer; we must live how we can. (*DH* 190-91)

The Death of the Heart is pitched on the threshold of the Second World War; it is a novel of inflexible middle-class manners and sensibilities soon to be shattered. Stilled, atrophied, the novel's slumbering pre-war London is haunted by an uncanny sense of its traumatic future. In this chapter, I read *The Death of the Heart* as a study of sleep as a psychophysiological and sociological response to trauma – as an exploration of "atrophy, not of death so much as of death sleep". In this novel, "death sleep" becomes a typically strange

[1] Bowen, "Elizabeth Bowen and Jocelyn Brooke in Conversation", 7.

and Bowenesque metaphor for anaesthetizing oneself to the past. *The Death of the Heart* suggests that to allow a part of the self to atrophy, to become numb, to go to sleep, is the only way one can go on living after trauma. As Eddie and St Quentin tell the adolescent Portia Quayne, "I've started to live in one way, because that's been the only way I can live" (*DH* 359). Atrophy, in this text, comes to imply an inability to cope with the traumatic event and integrate it into conscious thought. The "key to why people do what they do" is the key to the past, to those traumatic events and experiences locked away, put to sleep, in order for the self to survive (*ibid.*, 331). That which innocent Portia sees as falsehood is rather a protective layer for the traumatized psyche. Drawing on work by Caruth and by Jacqueline Rose, in relation to Freud's work on dreams, sleep, and awakening, this chapter uses the dream-work of *The Death of the Heart* and of Bowen's short story, "The Apple Tree" (1934) to consider the ways in which these narratives contribute to our ideas about the unconscious and the memory of trauma, and the relationship between trauma and survival.

In Freud's work, Rose points out, death and sleep "appear as vanishing points of psychoanalysis". She argues that at such points, "Freud appears to be telling, or rather showing, us that there are places in our mind and in our histories – in the histories he lived through – which even the idea of the unconscious is insufficient to grasp".[2] Sleep and death in Bowen's work point to a similar slipperiness with regard to the traumas of "our mind and … our histories". Indeed, in *The Death of the Heart*, death, sleep and dreams edge towards that ungraspable space of trauma outside "the real", and outside the realist text. The unknowability of death and sleep Rose notes in Freud's work can be tracked in *The Death of the Heart* through Matchett's reverence for her evening rituals, as she "served the idea of sleep with a series of little ceremonials" (*DH* 90). Matchett is so "in awe of approaching sleep" that she is reluctant even to acknowledge her own need to sleep or to show fatigue (*ibid.*, 90; see also 306, 382). By making "a sort of altar of each bed", the "monklike" (*ibid.*, 24) Matchett shows her worship for sleep, "the silent tide" (*ibid.*, 90). Bowen, Rose notes, is "particularly apt at showing how – beyond all

[2] Jacqueline Rose, *On Not Being Able to Sleep: Psychoanalysis and the Modern World*, London: Chatto and Windus, 2003, 8.

reason – perceptual boundaries between inner and outer worlds can break down".[3] In this way, death sleep in this novel mimics the liminal, or hypnagogic "nowhere" space between sleeping and waking, between remembering and forgetting. If it is true, as Rose suggests, that such "Barriers inside and between minds start to crumble when the world is falling apart", then the state of death sleep in *The Death of the Heart* can be seen as a traumatic anticipation of the war which would follow just a year after its publication.[4]

In *The Death of the Heart*, sixteen-year-old orphan Portia is uprooted from the nomadic existence she had lived with her parents and forced into the structure and routine of the stylish London home of her half-brother, Thomas, and his wife, Anna. Portia becomes romantically involved with Eddie (who is never graced with a surname), one of Anna's admirers – a situation that causes much concern, not only for Anna and Thomas, but for their housekeeper, Matchett, and their friends, Major Brutt and St Quentin Miller. When Portia's heart is ultimately broken by Eddie, and she also discovers that Anna has read her diary, she seeks solace in the bumbling Major Brutt, whom she believes to be "the same" as her: unsettled, uncertain, dependent upon the tolerance of others more fortunate (*DH* 380). The girl fails to return to Windsor Terrace by the end of the novel, and the reader is left, with Portia and Matchett, suspended on the threshold of Major Brutt's hotel. Portia's adolescent imitation of the adults' psychological behaviour points up their anaesthetization; in other words, Portia, "the awake one", "imparts meaning" for the death sleep of the novel's adults, especially Anna.

Anna-esthetics

Dwelling on the past and, especially, mourning, Anna believes, is a vice; when first confronted with a solemn and recently orphaned Portia she is quick to remove her black garments and outward signs of loss and memorialization, and "explained at once that mourning not only did not bring the dead back but did nobody good" (*ibid.*, 49). Anna has become numb to her traumatic past – her miscarried children, the death of her mother, the loss of her lover Robert Pidgeon – and she exemplifies the narrator's observation that, "We desert those

---

[3] *Ibid.*, 9.

[4] *Ibid.*, 106.

who desert us; we cannot afford to suffer; we must live how we can" (*ibid.*, 190-91). Anna is atrophied; she has "set" or frozen (*ibid.*, 31). Anna's forgetting, however, leaves her numb and scarred: her memory, traumatized, "was all blurs and seams" (*ibid.*, 53). The years she spent with Pidgeon are unreadable, "closed" to her (*idem*), and as Allan E. Austin points out, Anna "harbours Pidgeon in the recesses of her mind in the same way that she has his letters secreted in a secret drawer of her desk".[5] Portia's unexpected arrival exposes Anna's repression:

> But during the conversation about Pidgeon, Anna had felt [Portia's] dark eyes with a determined innocence steal back again and again to her face .... Anna felt bound up with her fear, with her secret, by that enwrapping look of Portia's: she felt mummified. (*DH* 58)

Anna is figured as an embalmed corpse, an already-dead body, wrapped and preserved. For Major Brutt, Pidgeon is "a big fly in the amber of [his] memory", stilled and stored while alive, and thus Anna becomes a vessel of dead memories, laid in the pose of death sleep (*ibid.*, 53). Foreshadowed by the frozen lake in Regent's Park on which the novel opens (*ibid.*, 3), Anna's smooth, hard surface conceals the tumult of dark waters beneath; she even speaks "with the perfect smoothness of ice" (*ibid.*, 394). At the height of winter Anna, like the bear whose fur she wears, hibernates.

Like Emmeline in *To the North*, Anna is also conceived of as physically still: she is like the waxworks at Madame Tussaud's where Portia and Eddie lunch, for "She could stay so still, and she so greatly disliked other people to fidget, that to fidget herself was almost an act of passion" (*ibid.*, 85). However, while Emmeline's stillness is symptomatic of a more profound, and unconscious, psychological detachment, Anna works to maintain her condition of stillness, her death sleep, as a psychophysiological defence. For Eddie, she is "one mass of pretence" (*ibid.*, 82). Thus, for example, Anna is anxious to assure St Quentin that she and Thomas are "not having a scene", so that the image of her life should not slip (*ibid.*, 396, 402). Thomas, too, acknowledges her performance when he tells her that "If you were half as heartless as you make out, you would be an appallingly

---

[5] Austin, *Elizabeth Bowen*, 59.

boring woman" (*ibid.*, 318). Indeed, Anna's heart is not absent, but a "turned-in heart", rather like a "shut-in room"; it is masked by "that specious mystery the individual throws about himself" (*ibid.*, 73).

> Having been seen at the window, having been waved to, made Anna step back instinctively. She knew how foolish a person looking out of a window appears from the outside of a house – as though waiting for something that does not happen, as though wanting something from the outside world. A face at a window for no reason is a face that should have a thumb in its mouth; there is something only-childish about it. (*Ibid.*, 321)

Anna's instinct is to retreat from "the outside world". The smooth façade of the house mirrors that of her face, a face that gives nothing away. "A face at a window" is the "thumb in its mouth" of the house, forlorn and vulnerable. Anna refuses to look as if she wants anything from another person, for in her experience, one loses all that one wants or loves. Anna's mask is a means of self-protection, a shield for the vulnerable little girl she remains.

Memory threatens Anna's anaesthetized present. As she is so fond of reciting, "experience means nothing till it repeats itself" (*ibid.*, 322), and Anna makes her experiences "nothing", insisting that Pidgeon "thought nothing" of her: "Nothing really happened" (*ibid.*, 346). Anna, observes Matchett, "would rather not have the past" (*ibid.*, 101). Her experience thus becomes what St Quentin describes as "These *lacunae* in people!" until she reads the repetition of that experience in Portia (*ibid.*, 330). The arrival of Portia – and, indeed, of Major Brutt ("the appendix to the finished story of Robert" [*ibid.*, 343]) – forces Anna to reread the past. Portia, like Leopold in *The House in Paris*, is the trace of that shameful past which "has to come back", the remains Anna is forced to read (*ibid.*, 99):

> Portia was not like Anna, already half-way through a woman's checked, puzzled life, a life to which the intelligence only gives a further distorted pattern. With Anna, feeling was by now unwilling, but she had more resonance. Memory enlarged and enlarged inside her an echoing, not often visited cave. Anna could remember being a child more easily and with more pleasure than she could remember being Portia's age: with her middle 'teens a cloudy phase had begun. She

> did not know half she remembered till a sensation touched her; she forgot to look back till these first evenings of spring. (*Ibid.*, 158-59)

Anna's habit of repression is, in this passage, a function of her gender, because a "woman's … life" is "checked" and "puzzled". Desires are scratched out, denied, so that instead, Anna harbours inside her an enlarging, empty cave. Anna's life as a woman is "checked" or marked by these patterns of forgetting, but it is also "checked" or stopped short, prevented from further growth. In "these first evenings of spring", the "sensation" of the past touches her through Portia's diary, rousing her repressed memories from their winter iciness.

More particularly, that repression or blurring began in her adolescence, the time when she, like Portia, lost her mother. The diary draws Anna back to this "cloudy phase" and forces her to reread and to relive the past (*ibid.*, 322). Thus, while her observation of Portia's adolescence reminds Anna of her own, more importantly the narrative is precipitated by her reading of Portia's diary, for that reading begins to shatter Anna's iciness, her determination to make "feeling … unwilling".[6] The arrival of Portia, daughter of the "leak[y]" (*ibid.*, 17) Irene, disrupts the careful constructed façade of life in the house on Windsor Terrace (not least when she spills ink on the white rug of her bedroom), but also melts the "brittle film" of Anna's icy defence (*ibid.*, 3). Indeed, as David Trotter has recognized, Anna finds the diary precisely because she is clearing up Portia's untidy bedroom – and more specifically, because Portia's failure to keep her papers, as Anna hoards her letters, locked away, makes Anna "shake with anger – I really can't tell you why" (*ibid.*, 6).[7] But this understanding of death sleep makes clear that Anna is angry because the textual space of the diary, like the *escritoire* in which it was kept, "gush[es]", abject, over its borders of privacy, forcing a confrontation between the past and the present, and moreover, forcing Anna's confrontation of her atrophy (*DH* 6). In this way, it might be said to instigate Anna's final "spilling over, the burst of tears and words, the ejaculation of the

[6] Anna explicitly compares Eddie and Portia to her own relationship with Pidgeon: "Directly the two had gone out after tea, she had gone to this drawer with the clearly recognized intention of comparing the falseness of Pidgeon with the falseness of Eddie" (*DH* 322).

[7] David Trotter, *Cooking with Mud: The Idea of Mess in Nineteenth-Century Art and Fiction*, Oxford: Oxford University Press, 2000, 6.

private personal grief" (*ibid.*, 355). That confrontation or "consummation" reaches its climax in the novel's final scenes, and leads Thomas to ask of Anna, "How much is the diary, how much is you?" (*ibid.*, 409-10).

The Quaynes' housekeeper, Matchett, recognizes that the past cannot be ignored; "Those without memories", she tells Portia, "don't know what is what" (*ibid.*, 99). She thus comes to represent for Portia not only an alternative figure of maternity, but of memory. Matchett and Portia, Anna says, "talk about the past":

> "The past?" said Thomas. "What do you mean? Why?"
> "Their great mutual past – your father, naturally."
> "What makes you think that?"
> "Their being so knit up. They sometimes look like each other. What other subject – except of course, love – gives people that sort of obsessed look? Talk like that is one climax the whole time. It's a trance; it's a vice; it's a sort of complete world." (*Ibid.*, 408)

For Anna, remembering is akin to living in a hypnotic inner world, an unhealthy fixation or a "vice". To be "obsessed" with the past, she says, is to be caught in "a trance": a kind of death sleep. Anna's insistence on a defence against the past figures a trance-like obsession. Just as Mr Quayne "had got knit up with Irene in a sort of dream wood", "knit up" in the obsession of romantic love (*ibid.*, 19), so too, Anna says, Portia and Matchett are "knit up" with each other, and "knit up" with the past, bound in a series of entrancing, hallucinatory knots. The past, she suggests, ensnares one.

By contrast, Matchett and Portia demonstrate that remembering, and therefore moving between past and present, is possible. Matchett facilitates this temporal interaction. She proffers the past to Portia, "as though her body were a vaseful of memory that must not be spilt" (*ibid.*, 95). In the novel's final scene, Matchett is the vessel of memory and narrator of the past; "with an air of authority", she is the precipitant of action beyond the confines of the text (*ibid.*, 418). As Hermione Lee has recognized, the novel's conclusion suggests that survival, moving forward into the future, will rely on an acknowledgement of the power of the past.[8]

---

[8] Lee, *Elizabeth Bowen*, 114.

Performing survival

Contemporary theories of traumatic memory are circumscribed by a concern with sleep and in particular, with sleep activity, such as dreaming. Indeed, for Caruth, Freud's *The Interpretation of Dreams* (1899) is preoccupied with this connection between trauma and sleep; over and over, she says, it asks, "*What does it mean to sleep? And what does it mean to wish to sleep?*" and moreover, "*What does it mean to awaken?*"[9] To wish to sleep, Freud suggests, figures a desire to escape an unsatisfactory reality and to, in dream, fulfil a wish "within the unconscious fantasy world of the psyche".[10] Portia's socialization rests on this literal and metaphorical belief in sleep as a refuge. No maternal figure in the novel – Anna, Matchett, Mrs Heccombe – encourages a type of sleep which, for Portia, described her life with her mother, their unity and pre-Oedipal symbiosis: "at nights [they] had pulled their beds close together or slept in the same bed – overcoming, as far as might be, the separation of birth." (*DH* 68-69) Now, when she prepares for sleep it is as if she is preparing for death, so that she lies "in a sort of coffin of silence" (*ibid.*, 105). In a room described as like a place in which a death has occurred (*ibid.*, 411), Portia obediently lies like a corpse, feigning sleep – indeed, feigning death sleep.

> Immediately, Portia shut her eyes, set her mouth and lay stiff on the pillow, as though so much light dug into a deep wound. She felt it must be very late, past midnight: that point where the river of night flows underneath time, that point at which occurs the mysterious birth of tomorrow. The very sudden, anaesthetic white light, striped by the pleats of the shade, created a sense of sickroom emergency. As though she lay in a sickroom, her spirit retreated to a seclusion of its own. (*Ibid.*, 105-106)

---

[9] Caruth, *Unclaimed Experience*, 97, 99; original emphasis. Caruth refers to a father who had fallen asleep shortly after the death of his son, and dreamed that the boy called to him, "Father, don't you see I'm burning?" Upon waking he saw that the man employed to watch over his child's corpse had also fallen asleep and allowed a candle to fall and set fire to the death shroud. To continue to sleep, in this case, would enable him to remain in the presence of his son, whose voice he had never thought to hear again; to awaken, however, permitted him to rescue the real body of his child. See Sigmund Freud, *The Interpretation of Dreams* (1899), trans. Joyce Crick, Oxford: Oxford University Press, 1999, 330-32.

[10] Caruth, *Unclaimed Experience*, 97.

Portia firmly shuts her eyes, refusing the light – waking reality – that threatens to penetrate and shine upon her "deep wound". However, the tentative language of the passage underscores that Portia does not actually retreat from her trauma, but here *plays* at death sleep; by mimicking the behaviour of those around her, she demonstrates her recognition of sleep as a performed anaesthesia or immunity. In this way, Portia attempts to fit into the stiff proprieties of this society, like Eddie, who also plays at death when he pretends to be a "lady's fox fur" and makes "himself look as if he had glass eyes, like a fur" (*ibid.*, 150). But most importantly, Portia "mim[es] sorrow – in fact, this immediate, this obedient prostration of her whole being was meant to hold off the worst, the full of grief, that might sweep her away" (*ibid.*, 98). The performance of grief divides Portia's affect from her inner turmoil. Portia acknowledges her sorrow, but like a child who mimics an adult in order to learn, her imitation of Anna's immunity begins with this division of the inner and outer selves. That is, she merely goes through the motions of affect, and so partitions her traumatic memory from its outward enactment. This is the point on which the novel turns, the meaning Portia imparts upon the other characters: Portia demonstrates the process of repressing traumatic events, and highlights why those around her are the way they are. She is the "key" to why these characters "do what they do".

Portia's wish to sleep, her wish for death sleep, is most overwhelming after the trauma of Eddie's betrayal. Thus, while Portia is figured as the novel's "awake" character, Eddie incites in her a "desire" for sleep that approaches Anna's response to Pidgeon:

> At the very sound, on Eddie's lips, of the word, desire to sleep had spread open inside Portia like a fan ....
>
> Since the talk with St Quentin, the idea of betrayal had been in her, upon her, sleeping and waking, as might be one's own guilt, making her not confront any face with candour, making her dread Eddie. Being able to shut her eyes while he was in this room with her, to feel impassive marble against her cheek, made her feel in the arms of immunity – the immunity of sleep, of anaesthesia, of endless solitude, the immunity of the journey across Switzerland two days after her mother died. She saw that tree she saw when the train stopped for no reason; she saw in her nerves, equally near and distant, the wet trees out there in the park. She heard the Seale sea, then heard the silent distances of the coast.

> There was a pause in the drawingroom. Then Anna said: "I wish I could just do that; I wish I were sixteen." (*Ibid.*, 336-37)

At Eddie's eerily hypnotic command to sleep, Portia feels the tug of slumber as an escape, underscoring Caruth's argument that, in Freud's work, the wish to sleep involves, in part, the desire to escape from reality. No longer performing, Portia adopts the coping mechanisms of those around her, and in particular, Anna; she has come to see sleep as an anaesthetic to the painful present, an escape from the knowledge of Eddie's betrayal that has disrupted her innocence. And when Portia discovers that betrayal has extended to the rest of the Windsor Terrace household, she flees to Major Brutt's hotel where, climbing into his bed, she enacts the defensive ritual of sleep: "folding her arms over [the eiderdown] tightly", she "lock[s]" it, "her last shelter, to her chest" (*ibid.*, 390).

Growing up, in *The Death of the Heart*, is paradoxical, for it does not suggest that with maturity comes an ability to adequately deal with trauma; rather, adulthood appears only to imply a greater aptitude for repression. The shedding of innocence in this novel thus occurs simultaneously to the process of atrophy. In this way, *The Death of the Heart* chronicles the death of childhood; to grow up, to become socialized, is to become numbed or immune to the pain of the adult. The "desire to sleep" does not only figure a wish for unconsciousness, but also describes the movement of Anna and Portia from desire, to sleep: from traumatic desire for Pidgeon and Eddie, to sleep or atrophy as a response to trauma.

Moreover if, as Freud posits, the wish to sleep is a motive for dream, Portia's desire to sleep may be seen as a desire to dream of, or to return to the past, a site of immunity from the present, prior to the traumatic event.[11] Significantly, the places to which she returns are liminal – a paused train, the coastline; she refuses to commit to any point of certainty, and in this way becomes immune to the flow of time and space. The "impassive marble" she rests against reassures her atrophy. Anna's stated wish to sleep – "I wish I could just do that; I wish I were sixteen" – also figures a desire to return to a time prior

---

[11] "*Thus the wish to sleep must always be included among the motives for the formation of dreams, and every successful dream is a fulfilment of that wish*" (Freud, *The Interpretation of Dreams*, 181; original emphasis).

to the traumatic event. For both women, the wish to sleep figures a wish to return to an idealized past, a liminal or "nowhere" space of false immunity. But more than this, Anna's desire to sleep suggests that she does not recognize that she is already subject to death sleep. Indeed, to acknowledge this would be to awaken. If, as Caruth suggests, to "awaken is thus to bear the imperative to survive", death sleep is false survival.[12] Atrophy, living how one can, is not survival, but a performance of it, a performance exposed by the mimic, Portia.

"Dream wood"

Death sleep is first figured as a response to trauma in Bowen's short story, "The Apple Tree", published four years prior to *The Death of the Heart*. Myra is the new, young wife of Simon Wing, who hosts a weekend party for several of his friends. Myra's somnambulist activity disturbs several guests, who subsequently discover that the girl regularly suffers the memory or hallucination of her discovery of a school friend who had committed suicide in the large apple tree of the school grounds. "The Apple Tree" is, like *The Death of the Heart*, a narrative concerned with sleep and anaesthesia: the Wings' guests struggle against "numbing feet and spines creeping" during a cold, dull local concert; later, Lancelot observes that "the return to Simon of sensibility and intelligence, like circulation beginning again in a limb that had been tightly bound up, was too much for Simon" – he faints, falling unconscious to the floor.[13] Lancelot, ironically, cannot sleep: "The very comfort of bed, the too exquisite sympathy with his body of springs and mattress, became oppressive .... With jealousy and nostalgia he pictured them all asleep. Mrs Wing's cheek would scarcely warm a pillow" ("AT" 463). The oppressive bed is, as in *The Death of the Heart*, like a swaddling coffin. Lancelot's "jealousy and nostalgia" of his sleeping friends foreshadows Anna's envy of Portia, while the coldness of Myra's cheek likens her to a corpse; the girl, like Portia, mimics death sleep in an attempt to hold off traumatic return, as "Flattening among the bedclothes, she tried hard to obliterate herself" (*ibid.*, 467), and she lies with her "eyes shut, cheek pressed to

---

[12] Caruth, *Unclaimed Experience*, 105.

[13] Elizabeth Bowen, "The Apple Tree" (1934), in *Collected Stories*, 461, 465. Hereafter cited parenthetically as "AT".

the pillow as though she were sleeping, but with her body rigid" (*ibid.*, 468).

Myra's dreams exemplify the Freudian compulsion to repeat. For Myra, sleep has become entwined with death; ever since the first night her sleep was disturbed by the discovery of her friend's suicide, the experience has been repeated. "The strongest compulsions we feel throughout life are no more than compulsions to repeat a pattern: the pattern is not of our own device", *The Death of the Heart* asserts, in a peculiarly Freudian manner (*DH* 219). Myra is unable to consciously assimilate her friend's death – perhaps due to a sense of her own guilt, for she had earlier told Doria that she "wished she was dead" ("AT" 469). This guilt, Lassner suggests, "has stilted her development", and means that both she (a "mannerless, sexless child" [*ibid.*, 463]) and Doria "remain children, one in death and the other in life".[14] Now, Myra is compelled, night after night, to repeat the traumatic discovery. She recalls:

> She and I still slept in the same room, with two others. That night – there was some moon – I saw her get up. She tied the cord of her dressing-gown – it was very thick – round her waist tightly; she looked once at me, but I pretended to be asleep. I lay – there was only a little moon – with a terrible feeling, like something tight round my throat. ("AT" 469)

Myra's punishment for stillness, for feigning sleep, is to be trapped in this dream, in this death sleep; sleep-walking, she behaves as if she were awake, but is caught in sleep, sentenced to traumatic repetition. The "terrible feeling" of "something tight round [her] throat" unconsciously identifies the weapon Doria will use to take her own life, as well as figuring the recognizably frustrating atrophy and mutism of dream-reality. In the stammering parentheses of the text, again and again, Myra fails to cry out to save her friend.

This story anticipates Portia's dream, which presents Anna, like Myra, as "an absolute child", emotionally atrophied (*ibid.*, 461). Although Portia is frequently shown lying in bed, she is never asleep – even late at night, when she is expected to be deep in slumber, she

---

[14] Phyllis Lassner, *Elizabeth Bowen: A Study of the Short Fiction*, New York, Twayne, 1991, 50, 51.

whispers to a concerned Matchett, "I'm awake" (*DH* 90). The one exception to this occurs on Portia's first night away from London, when she experiences an unusual dream.[15]

> Portia dreamed she was sharing a book with a little girl. The tips of Anna's long fair hair brushed on the page: they sat up high in a window, waiting till something happened. The worst of all would be if the bell rang, and their best hope was to read to a certain point in the book. But Portia found she no longer knew how to read – she did not dare tell Anna, who kept turning pages over. She knew they must both read – so the fall of Anna's hair filled her with despair, pity, for what would have to come. The forest (there was a forest under the window) was being varnished all over: it left no way of escape. (*DH* 181)

In this dream, Anna never acknowledges Portia's presence; Portia, on the other hand, is shown to be hyper-aware of her surroundings. She is alert to something about to happen, unlike the young Anna who "kept turning pages over". Again, Anna is shown to be numb to, or shut off from, the world, while Portia is awake. Both, however, are still, waiting; they are like Rapunzel in her tower, alike even in the swing of Anna's "mimosa yellow" hair (*ibid.*, 182). The text also stresses the interaction of the dream world and waking reality, for Portia realizes that "worst of all would be if the bell rang" and in this way incorporates the possibility of bells or an alarm into her dream, thus guarding her sleep by defending herself against the reality of an alarm clock waking her up.[16] Anna later touches on this desire, imagining that Portia feels a "Wish that someone outside would blow a whistle and make the whole thing stop", that the novel's adults would awaken, their fantastic fictions of lives thwarted (*DH* 409).

When Portia does wake up the reader is privy to her hypnagogic state, "the haunted outer court of the dream" (*ibid.*, 182). The voices Portia awakens to, "like whispers down the clinic corridor, or sounds in the forest still left from the dream", do not only spill across this

---

[15] The dream of a forest recurs in Bowen's only children's book, *The Good Tiger* (1965); the tiger dreams "he was a baby tiger once more. All round were trees, bright green trees, and the sun was hot. In his dream, the tiger knew where he was. This was the forest, his own forest. In his dream, the tiger hopped and jumped" (London: Jonathan Cape, 1970, n.p.).

[16] Freud, *The Interpretation of Dreams*, 26.

hypnagogic boundary, but recall her earlier thought that sleep is like being in a "sickroom" (*ibid*., 181). The forest of Portia's dream is the most striking hallucinatory image here, for this forest does not only recreate the "dream wood" of her parents' early romance, but becomes atrophied wood of the type that can be "varnished". This type of wood is impenetrable – "it left no way of escape". The dream is thus a false hope: sleep is not an escape but merely a means of postponing "what would have to come", the inevitable plot of the narrative the girls share. The only way out of the dream is not through the window or the forest, but through a traumatic awakening. This dream is revelatory for Portia, for it not only enables her to recognize Anna's vulnerability, but awakens her to the futility of death sleep and of repressing trauma. The dream reveals to Portia the "unknowing sorrow" (*ibid*., 270) Anna hides behind her curtain of hair, and the realization that Anna, too, "sometimes, [did] not know what to do next" (*ibid*., 182). "Inside everyone", Portia now wonders, "is there an anxious person who stands to hesitate in an empty room?" (*ibid*., 182).

The novel's adult characters advocate a censorship which Portia at first resists, but to which she gradually learns to adhere. Her insistence upon leaving in her diary a blank page to represent those days on which she had nothing to write points up her reluctance to forget that a day had occurred, yet this empty space and the repression it signals is just as telling as anything she might choose to write. Eddie pushes her to censor him from her diary, and therefore to undertake the editing and cloaking of memory that the novel's adults carry out. St Quentin, for example, "edits memory in order to transform reality into a tolerable fiction", and Eddie's libellous novel directly draws fiction from life.[17] Censorship, in his satirical novel, is only superficially exercised, and Eddie is (socially) punished. He suggests to Portia his inability to differentiate between life and fiction when he tells her, "Plot – It's a revolution: it's our life. The whole pack are against us. So hide, hide everything" (*DH* 129), and "I really do quite like Anna. But we have got to have a villain of some sort" (*ibid*., 132). Not only does Eddie apply too little indiscretion to his writing of life, but he assumes that the rules of narrative are also relevant to life. Indeed, Eddie is himself a fiction, a "pantomime" shielding a "vacuum" (*ibid*., 82).

[17] Lassner, *Elizabeth Bowen*, 110.

However, the novelist, St Quentin, advocates a distinction between fact and fiction, and encourages Portia's textual and personal censorship:

> I should never write what had happened down. One's nature is to forget, and one ought to go by that. Memory is quite unbearable enough, but even so it leaves out quite a lot. It wouldn't let one down as gently, even, as that if it weren't more than half a fake – we remember to suit ourselves. No, really, er, Portia, believe me: if one didn't let oneself swallow some few lies, I don't know how one would ever carry the past .... But a diary (if one did keep it up to date) would come much too near the mark. One ought to secrete for sometime before one begins to look back at anything. Look how reconciled to everything reminiscences are .... Also, suppose somebody read it? (*Ibid.*, 327)

St Quentin perceives that writing a diary overcomes the "natur[al]" tendency of memory to "forget", to "fake", to protect. Memory, he suggests, is fiction, a varnished illusion, a dream wood. To "secrete" such varnish, such falsity, is a defence which enables "reconcil[iation]" and survival. Moreover, insofar as Portia's diary is the precipitant for the narrative's action, St Quentin's final question points up a concern not for the protection of its author's secrets, but for its effect upon the reader of the diary (that is, Anna), exposed to Portia's raw narration.

In *The Death of the Heart*, the coping mechanisms of the novel's adults encourage Portia's anaesthetization to trauma as the only socially acceptable form of survival; her subsequent performance of grief demonstrates the beginning of her socialization and her initial movement from the free emotion of childhood to a constrained, atrophied adulthood. Although the girl attempts to remove herself from such influence, at the novel's end the adolescent Portia remains suspended in this liminal state, caught at a crossroads of alternative adult models and alternative memory practices.

CHAPTER 5

SAFE: WARTIME SHORT FICTION

> The hallucinations in the stories are not a peril; nor are the stories studies of mental peril. The hallucinations are an unconscious, instinctive, saving resort on the part of the characters: life, mechanized by the controls of wartime, and emotionally torn and impoverished by changes, had to complete itself in *some* way.[1]

> Outwardly, we were of course prepared to support the view that death is the inevitable outcome of all life, that each of us owes nature a death and must be prepared to settle the debt, in short, that death is natural, undeniable and inevitable. In reality, however, we tend to behave as though things were otherwise. We have shown the unmistakable tendency to push death aside, to eliminate it from life. We have tried to keep it deadly silent; … fundamentally no one believes in his own death or, which comes to the same thing: in the unconscious each of us is convinced of his immortality.[2]

The fantasy of immortality is a "saving resort", a "saving hallucination".[3] Wartime illusions, Bowen suggests, compensate for an "impoverished" reality, for the kind of "meaner living" I discussed in the Introduction to this book. Consoling, they form an evening balm for the traumatic wounds and ruptures of the heat of the day. But more than this, the short stories Bowen wrote during the Second World War, published in *The Demon Lover and Other Stories* and *Look At All Those Roses and Other Stories*, explore the ways in which unconscious fantasies become a site of escape from the present, in

[1] Elizabeth Bowen, "Postscript to *The Demon Lover and Other Stories*" (1945), in *The Mulberry Tree*, 96 (original emphasis).
[2] Sigmund Freud, "Timely Reflections on War and Death" (1915), in *On Murder, Mourning and Melancholia*, trans. Shaun Whiteside, London: Penguin, 2005, 183.
[3] Bowen, "Postscript to *The Demon Lover*", 96, 97.

which death can no longer be kept "deadly silent". Just as Londoners were each night during the Blitz forced underground for protection, in these stories retreat into psychical recesses is necessary for survival. In order "To save something" – to protect, to hoard, and to survive – civilians, like the city itself, were forced to "[contract] round [their] wounds".[4]

In this chapter I argue that Bowen's wartime short stories posit hallucination, or life lived within the unconscious, not as a representation of trauma, terror or sadness, but rather of protection and safety. Whereas elsewhere in Bowen's fiction psychological detachment problematizes identity and narrative, in her wartime short fiction it figures a kind of psychical defence of these. The psychic savings enable the characters of these stories to except themselves, and to be kept safe, from the traumatic reality of war.[5] "We all lived in a state of lucid abnormality", Bowen later recalled, suggesting that wartime civilians lived in a state of lucid dream, living on, surviving, in the safety of an unconscious unable to imagine its own non-existence.[6] This means that Bowen's wartime short fiction testifies to a Freudian refusal of death. Psychic retreat into the safety and, indeed, the safe of one's unconscious in these stories figures the imperative to "live how one can" – it figures the human desire for survival.

Infected Ireland

For Derrida, the "safe" is interchangeable with the "crypt"; the "inner safe", for example, also describes the traumatic crypt.[7] As Barbara Johnson points out in her translation of the essay of the same name, *fors* is, "in French, derived from the Latin *foris* ('outside, outdoors'),

---

[4] Elizabeth Bowen, "London, 1940" (1950), in *The Mulberry Tree*, 23.

[5] Gill Plain has noted that escape for Bowen's wartime characters may be in terms of "a space which rejects the temporal order of war, and enables them to spiritually abscond from the physical environment of conflict. These defences against the disruptions and chaos of war leave the characters emotionally isolated and distanced from their environment, but in Bowen's work alienation is frequently presented as an essential prerequisite of survival" (*Women's Fiction of the Second World War: Gender, Power and Resistance*, Edinburgh: Edinburgh University Press, 1996, 122).

[6] Bowen, "Postscript to *The Demon Lover*", 95.

[7] Jacques Derrida, "*Fors*: The Anglish Words of Nicolas Abraham and Maria Torok", trans. Barbara Johnson, in Nicolas Abraham and Maria Torok, *The Wolf Man's Magic Word: A Cryptonomy*, trans. Nicholas T. Rand (1976), Minneapolis: University of Minnesota Press, 1986, xi-xlviii.

[and] is an archaic preposition meaning 'except for, barring, save'".[8] In terms of the way in which the melancholic subject psychologically incorporates the lost love object, Johnson here refers to the idea that the loved one has been lost, "save" inside me; they are dead, absent, "except for" in my unconscious.[9] This same desire to "push death aside" appears in Bowen's wartime short fiction, not as a melancholic inability to cope with loss, but rather as a manifestation of the will to survive: "an unconscious, instinctive, saving resort." If it is true, as Freud points out, that war fails to keep the pact of "deadly silen[ce]", the wartime potential for loss and for death provokes in Bowen's short fiction a kind of incorporation of the self. That is, mortality is made explicit everywhere "save" in the unconscious. And if, for Derrida, "the crypt is the vault of a desire", then in these stories, that desire is for the survival of the self.[10] In this way, the psyche becomes a kind of safe that enables survival. Under the relentless rain of bombing, and in the suffocating midst of an overcrowded city in which "they would even grudge you sharing a grave", the psychic safe might also represent a desire to preserve a small space of one's own.[11] In this chapter I examine Bowen's wartime stories, "impressions that stored themselves up and acquired force" until their release was commissioned.[12] In particular, "Summer Night", "Sunday Afternoon", and "The Happy Autumn Fields" bear witness to this desire to save and to be safe.

The wartime short stories of *The Demon Lover* and *Look At All Those Roses* not only guard against a threatening present; indeed, as Edwin J. Kenney has noted, even as these stories "show, in the face of the extremity of actual catastrophe, the instinctive and great power of

---

[8] Barbara Johnson, "Translator's Note to Derrida, '*Fors*'", in *The Wolf Man's Magic Word*, xi-xii.

[9] For further discussion of melancholic incorporation, see Abraham and Torok, "Mourning *or* Melancholia: Introjection *versus* Incorporation" (1972), in *The Shell and the Kernel*, 125-38.

[10] Derrida, "*Fors*", xvii.

[11] Elizabeth Bowen, "Mysterious Kôr" (1944), in *Collected Stories*, 731. Hereafter cited parenthetically as "MK".

[12] Bowen, "Postscript to *The Demon Lover*", 99. Requests for short fiction during the war, Bowen states, "acted as releases. Each time I sat down to write a story I opened a door; and the pressure against the other side of that door must have been very great, for things – ideas, images, emotions – came through with force and rapidity, sometimes violence" (*ibid.*, 94-95).

the human imagination to create and sustain new images of peace and immunity that allow life to go on", they also recreate "the childhood apprehension that nothing is safe".[13] "The Inherited Clock" (1944), for example, is concerned with the repetition of childhood trauma during a second global war. Here and elsewhere in Bowen's fiction, the metaphoric artillery of the "past" – that is, the First World War – "discharges its load of feeling into the anaesthetized and bewildered present".[14] Thus the act of remembering with which the story opens ("Yes, I can see you now"), has explosive consequences for the "anaesthetized and bewildered" Clara, who has repressed her childhood experience of the eerily named "skeleton clock".[15] But inheritance of the clock and of the past cannot be refused, however much Clara wishes to submit it to "annihilation" (*ibid.*, 635). It falls to Clara's co-inheritor, her cousin Paul, to recognize that, "*Your* trouble seems to be that you are stuck on the past" (*ibid.*, 636; original emphasis). In his retelling, his repetition, and his re-enactment of the traumatic event – luring Clara with the promise that she could hold a minute in her hand, he had forced the girl's finger into the cogs of the clock until it was crushed – the story demonstrates at once the compulsion to repeat an earlier trauma and suggests the shift from traumatic memory to narrative memory.[16] But even as the story's conclusion seems to suggest resolution, so that Clara is now able to "sit with my memories" ("IC" 640), Paul's earlier perception that "If you *have* forgotten, you must have some rather too good reason", makes the possibility of such resolution tenuous (*ibid.*, 636; original emphasis). Paul's insistence that he cannot take the clock thus figures a repetition of his "cruel tricks" (*ibid.*, 624). One is not so easily safe from trauma.

Other stories in *The Demon Lover* are more explicit about the traumatic return of the First World War; as Jordan notes, several of Bowen's characters in these stories respond "to the dislocations and shocks of the Second World War by reliving the enduring losses of the

---

[13] Kenney, *Elizabeth Bowen*, 65-66.

[14] Bowen, "Postscript to *The Demon Lover*", 98.

[15] Elizabeth Bowen, "The Inherited Clock" (1944), in *Collected Stories*, 623. Hereafter cited parenthetically as "IC".

[16] See Shafquat Towheed, "Territory, Space, Modernity: Elizabeth Bowen's *The Demon Lover and Other Stories* and Wartime London", in *Elizabeth Bowen: New Critical Perspectives*, ed. Susan Osborn, Cork: Cork University Press, 2009, 124.

previous world war".[17] Thus in "The Demon Lover" (1941), Kathleen Drover, who has briefly returned from the country to collect some items from her home in devastated London, finds a mysterious unstamped letter, appearing to be from her first fiancé, a soldier killed in the First World War, now demanding a rendezvous. In this story, the demon is an allegory for war: "in the midst of one war, a relic from an earlier one that was to have been the war to end all wars, would be a ghastly symbol of endless, inescapable violence."[18]

A fear that these traumatic cycles will never end is also expressed in "Ivy Gripped the Steps" (1945). This story is structured by the legacy of the last war, as during the Second World War Gavin, "too young for the last war, too old for this", revisits the house at Southstone where he had stayed as the clouds of the First World War loomed:[19]

> It was an existence mortgaged to necessity; it was an inheritance of uneasiness, tension and suspicion .... It was this dead weight of existence that had supplied to history not so much the violence or the futility ... but its repetitive harshness and its power to scar. This existence had no volition, but could not stop; and its never stopping, because it could not, made history's ever stopping the less likely. (*Ibid.*, 697)

In this story, "meaner living" has passed from impoverishment to a "mortgaged" existence that echoes the "debt" to nature – death – that Freud asserts we must be "prepared to settle". The human will to survive has become the "dead weight of existence", an existence that has no "volition", no will of its own, but clings to life like the tenacious and "tomb-defying" parasitic ivy (*ibid.*, 708). Moreover, it is, paradoxically, this very tenacity that has supplied history with "its

---

[17] Jordan, *How Will the Heart Endure*, 133.

[18] W.J. McCormack, "Irish Gothic and After (1820-1945)", in *The Field Day Anthology of Irish Writing*, ed. Seamus Deane, Derry: Field Day, 1991, II, 840. See also Daniel V. Fraustino, "Elizabeth Bowen's 'The Demon Lover': Psychosis or Seduction?", *Studies in Short Fiction*, XVII/4 (Fall 1980), 485; and Robert L. Calder, "'A More Sinister Troth': Elizabeth Bowen's 'The Demon Lover' as Allegory", *Studies in Short Fiction*, XXXI/1 (Winter 1994), 91-97.

[19] Elizabeth Bowen, "Ivy Gripped the Steps" (1945), in *Collected Stories*, 711. Hereafter cited parenthetically as "IGS".

repetitive harshness and its power to scar"; survival necessarily entails such traumatic effects.

"A Love Story: 1939" (1941), the first of Bowen's short stories explicitly situated during the Second World War, also draws on the influence of World War I. In this story, an exchange between a hotel's receptionist and a guest concerns war's reawakened presence:

> "But I tell you what – Were you never in the last war?" – "I was," said Frank. "But I'm not in this one, thank God." – "Now Miss Heally thought you had some military rank."[20]

The outbreak of war is at first ignored by the inhabitants of the small hotel in Ireland, as the "unheard news" of another disaster projects into an empty room (*ibid.*, 497). Indeed, the war is not made explicit until some way into the story: Clifford (later claimed to be the uncanny double, the repetition, of Mrs Massey's son, "a hero" [*ibid.*, 509]) and Polly Perry-Dunton "had been over here on honeymoon when the war began; here they still were, because of the war" (*ibid.*, 500); sequestering themselves from the threat, "they stayed on here where they were hidden and easy" (*ibid.*, 501).

In fact, throughout her wartime fiction, Bowen constructs Ireland as a space of refuge, a "neutral island" located beyond an embattled Europe.[21] Yet, Ireland does not only appear as a physical site of neutrality, but as a psychic symbolization of safety. Thus, while in "Sunday Afternoon", removal to Ireland represents a literal escape from the theatre of war, in "The Happy Autumn Fields", the latest story of the three explored here, and the one most embedded in the zone of wartime, escape is a fantasy and Ireland represents a region of safety for the psyche desperate for survival. However, the hallucinations of these stories represent more than a yearning to escape the danger and trauma of a war-torn present: such illusions actively seek survival. Psychical and physical Ireland is a neutral haven, a site of safety secluded from the "zone of death".[22] In

[20] Elizabeth Bowen, "A Love Story: 1939" (1941), in *Collected Stories*, 503. Hereafter cited parenthetically as "LS".

[21] This term is the title for Clair Wills' study: *That Neutral Island: A Cultural History of Ireland during the Second World War*, London: Faber and Faber, 2007.

[22] Elizabeth Bowen, "Sunday Afternoon" (1941), in *Collected Stories*, 621. Hereafter cited parenthetically as "SA".

"Summer Night", on the other hand, Ireland too is part of the "infected zone".[23] Set against the backdrop of the Battle of Britain – "An awful air battle. Destroying each other" – in this story the drone of fighter planes in the darkening sky makes a mockery of neutral Ireland's safety (*ibid.*, 585). Disillusion, disappointment, and death have spread. Yet, this story resists the admission of mortality. That is, even as "Summer Night" draws attention to the failure of some kinds of illusion, it maintains a site of wilful survival in Vivie, the child who bears the name of life.

"Summer Night" follows three narrative strands: Emma drives quickly through the Irish countryside, having left her family for the night in order to visit her lover, Robinson. Interspersed with Emma's journey are fragments of Robinson's evening, shared with two exhausting visitors, Justin Cavey, and his deaf sister, Queenie, as well as glimpses of Emma's home – of her two restless young daughters, her husband, the Major, and his anxious Aunt Fran. An atmosphere of shattered illusion, of impending danger, and of restlessness infects all three strands of the narrative: Justin and Robinson discuss the impossibility of thought under the pressure of war; Emma's daughter, Vivie, unable to sleep, runs riotously naked through the house; Aunt Fran prowls the corridors, watching for an unknown terror. Only Queenie remains calm, blissful in a private world of romantic memories. By the story's end, each of its strands has been disrupted by the encroaching threat of war, and each character has been confronted by the failures of their own illusions, save for Queenie, on whose drift into sleep the story ends.[24]

Most critics of the story have addressed it in terms of fairy-tales disturbed and romantic dreams shattered. Jeanette Shumaker, for example, considers the story as a binary relationship between Emma and Queenie, and their romantic illusions.[25] The latter, she argues, "does not want to be rescued" from the dream-memory of her fairy-tale lover, locked safe in her own world, while Emma desires "a

---

[23] Elizabeth Bowen, "Summer Night" (1941), in *Collected Stories*, 599. Hereafter cited parenthetically as "SN".

[24] Jeslyn Medoff, "'There is No Elsewhere': Elizabeth Bowen's Perceptions of War", *Modern Fiction Studies* XXX/1 (Spring 1984), 76.

[25] Jeanette Shumaker, "Bruised Boys and 'Fallen' Women: The Need for Rescue in Short Stories by Elizabeth Bowen", *South Carolina Review*, XXXII/1 (Fall 1999), 88-98. See also Lassner, *A Study of the Short Fiction*, 104.

saviour". Although the latter "discovers that her lover can't or won't rescue her", Shumaker adds, "she takes no steps to save herself".[26] Emma's romantic ideals and her "fairytale" are "broken", but not her heart ("SN" 605). For Shumaker, at least, the story's conceptualization of rescue, of safety, is an illusion of romantic love. Yet, Queenie's romanticism is not so self-serving. That is, Justin perceives her silence, and moreover, her immersion in memory as a means of ensnaring and suffocating him, rather than as her own space of romantic illusion or safety:

> He was down here with Queenie this summer only because of the war, which had locked him in: duty seemed to him better than failed pleasure .... His holiday with his sister, his holiday in this underwater, weedy region of memory, his holiday on which, almost every day, he had to pass the doors of their old home, threatened Justin with a pressure he could not bear. He had to share with Queenie, as he shared the dolls' house meals cooked on the oil stove behind her sitting-room screen, the solitary and almost fairylike world created by her deafness. Her deafness broke down his only defence, talk. He was exposed to the odd, immune, plumbing looks she was for ever passing over his face. (*Ibid.*, 587)

For Justin, a forced holiday in Ireland is synonymous with a "holiday in this underwater, weedy region of memory": not a site of refuge, but of the choking, entangling past. His "only defence, talk" is made useless by his sister's deafness, her "immun[ity]"; "exposed" to attack, his mind is "plumb[ed]", as if Queenie seeks to dredge Justin's own "weedy" psychical depths. And insofar as Queenie's "sphere of silence" is not described by language – "not a word clouded" it – her "fairylike world" of the past cannot be narrated, for it is outside "talk", outside the "word" (*ibid.*, 607). She thus makes talk, Justin's "defence" against or distraction from memory and wartime trauma, futile: "Above all, he was glad, for these hours or two of chatter [with Robinson], not to have to face the screen of his own mind, on which the distortion of every one of his images, the war-broken towers of Europe, constantly stood" (*ibid.*, 588). The very silence of Queenie, of Ireland, and of the past, applies its own wartime pressure.

---

[26] Shumaker, "Bruised Boys and 'Fallen' Women", 90, 92.

Furthermore, Queenie embodies the past, not only in terms of her continuation of Justin's childhood as she cooks for her brother "dolls' house meals", but also in her absorption in the memory of an earlier romance. Although Jordan states that "Queenie withdraws into the memory of a July night twenty years before",[27] it seems that Queenie's vision of the past is not a refuge, but rather threatens to encroach upon the present, putting it in danger of collapse:

> Queenie saw with joy in her own mind what she could not from her place in the window see – the blue china house, with all its reflecting windows, perched on its knoll in the brilliant, fading air. They are too rare – visions of where we are. ("SN" 591)

Although it is possible that Queenie here envisions the house as it might be seen by a spectator at that moment, in the act of remembering the house not as it is but as it was, she figures not just a spatial but a temporal survival of the past. This is reinforced by her later replacement of Robinson's face with that of the lover she had once walked with in the gardens:

> This was the night she knew she would find again. It had stayed living under a film of time. On just such a summer night, once only, she had walked with a lover in the demesne .... The subtle deaf girl had made the transposition of this nothing or everything into an everything – the delicate deaf girl that the man could not speak to and was afraid to touch. She who, then so deeply contented, kept in her senses each frond and breath of that night, never saw him again and had soon forgotten his face. That had been twenty years ago, till tonight when it was now. Tonight it was Robinson who, guided by Queenie down leaf tunnels, took the place on the stone seat by the lake. (*Ibid.*, 607-608)

Queenie refuses to accept the loss of her lover by ensuring that this one night "stayed living under a film of time". That night survives, safe in her memory, and enables Queenie to "[stay] living" by screening the blissful past over the traumatic present. Her memory, the point on which the story concludes, thus serves as a counter-attack against this disturbed wartime night, raiding, robbing and "plumbing" the present in order to ensure the survival of the past. And while for

[27] Jordan, *How Will the Heart Endure*, 145.

Aunt Fran war and death are inescapable – "There is not even the past: our memories share with us the infected zone; not a memory does not lead up to this. Every moment is everywhere, it holds the war in its crystal; there is no elsewhere, no other place" (*ibid.*, 599) – for Queenie, such temporal collapse ("it was now") is a means of living how she can.[28] By enabling the face of her past lover to be filled by a face in the present, by making "Every moment … everywhere", Queenie enables her lover's survival.

In his discussion of war and death, Freud posits that there are two central "factors responsible for the psychical distress of those who have remained at home … the disillusion that this war has provoked, and the altered attitude towards death which – like all other wars – it forces upon us".[29] As such, I now turn to the "psychical distress[es]" of "Summer Night", and in particular, Emma's "attitude towards death". As the darkness of the summer night draws closer to Emma's home, she telephones to wish her family a repeated "good night": "I just thought I'd say good night." ("SN" 593) In the iterations of this phrase, however, lies a latent admission of death. Despite her effort to construct a veiling illusion, Emma's embattled "good night" betrays her; it suggests, as Freud states, that "Death can now no longer be denied; we are obliged to believe in it".[30] "Good night", Royle argues:

> [is] the epitome of the colloquial: any and everyone can say it. The phrase is so conventional, so familiar, it doesn't require a second's reflection. And yet, it belongs to the liminal, belongs without belonging, at and as the very border: has "night" ever quite begun when one says "good night"? Strange "object" of a performative, when will it have begun? In particular as a so-called euphemism for "death" ("die well," "happy death," "have a good death now"), it

[28] The language of this passage echoes Bowen's description (written around the same time) of Bowen's Court as a wartime illusory "picture of peace": "Bowen's Court, in that December of 1941 in which this book was finished, still stood in its particular island of quietness, in the south of an island country not at war .... It was always with some qualification – most often with that of an almost undue joy – that one beheld, at Bowen's Court, the picture of peace. Looking, for instance, across the country from the steps in the evening, one thought: '*Can* pain and danger exist?' But one did think that. Why? The scene was a crystal in which, while one was looking, a shadow formed" (*BC* 456-57; original emphasis).

[29] Freud, "Timely Reflections on War and Death", 169.

[30] *Ibid.*, 185.

> names the unthinkable. But this unthinkable haunts every "good night." "Good night" is mad.[31]

In one way, Emma seems to seek from her husband, the Major, relic of and named by the last war, reassurance that the night is, indeed "good", in another mutation of the phrase, "It's a lovely night" ("SN" 593). Yet, her phone call is also an attempt to hide the "unthinkable" that "haunts" her "good night" – the possibility, that is, that she will not return – and her slippage from "It's a lovely night" to "It's a lovely night, isn't it?" points up her desire for her husband to maintain the illusion. Aunt Fran, however, does not play the game:

> "What's happened?"
> "Nothing. She rang up to say good night."
> "But she had said good night," said Aunt Fran in her troubled way. "She said good night to us when she was in the car. You remember, it was nearly night when she left. It seemed late to be starting to go so far. She had the whole afternoon, but she kept putting off, putting off. She seemed to me undecided up to the very last." (*Ibid.*, 594)

Aunt Fran recognizes Emma's "good night" as a strange, liminal phrase unable to define its limits and thus encroaching upon the night-time rituals of the house: tucking children into bed, closing and locking doors and windows. For Aunt Fran, disillusionment takes the form of revelation, as she recognizes that Emma's message is tainted or haunted by guilt. Emma's telephoned "good night" penetrates the security Aunt Fran has so anxiously desired: "She could begin to feel calmer now that the house was a fortress against the wakeful night" (*ibid.*, 595). That is, although her "good night" is, like Aunt Fran's prayers, ostensibly a wish for safety, for untroubled sleep, its surprising interruption of the household, as well as its unnecessary repetition, unsettles the old woman. Emma's uncertainty about when the night begins, and her inability to allow it to do so – wishing for "more time", as she does with Robinson, for with every "good night" the night begins, in a sense, again – points up her attempt to refuse the "unthinkable" and to keep darkness and death at bay, to "push death aside" (*ibid.*, 604).

[31] Nicholas Royle, *The Uncanny*, Manchester: Manchester University Press, 2003, 127.

The Major's termination of the phone call on the expression of yet another "Good night" and his sole performance of the household's evening rituals – for it is he alone who shuts, locks, and tucks – demonstrates that for him, the traumatic potential of darkness and death is best worked firmly against, and not permitted to lurk in the latent silences of unthinkability. Emma's "good night" is haunted by the unthinkableness of "nothing" happening, an unnamed silence that in part drives Aunt Fran's expostulation:

> It's never me, never me, never me! Whatever *I* see, whatever I hear it's "nothing," though the house might fall down. You keep everything back from me .... I am never told, never told, never told. I get the one answer, "nothing." (*Ibid.*, 597; original emphasis)

Aunt Fran refuses the illusion of safety constructed by the Major, his assertion that "nothing" threatens the security of the house, and that "nothing" is the reason Emma telephoned. As Aunt Fran seems to suspect, Emma's disturbing "good night" is the "Something" that has "got in" (*ibid.*, 597), the "something" that "will happen" (*ibid.*, 596). Indeed, what has "got in" is an admission of death. After Emma's telephone call, the living room "already felt the touch of decay; it threw lifeless reflections into the two mirrors" (*ibid.*, 597), enclosing Aunt Fran's "stranded", gasping body "like some object on the bed of a pool that has run dry" (*ibid.*, 594).[32] The Major's self-assurance of his family's safety – "He thought: it's all right, I locked the house" – cannot work against this infiltration (*ibid.*, 597).

Justin, too, bids Robinson "good night" in a letter to his host later that night:

> I wish you good night. Delicacy does not deter me from adding that I feel my good wish to be superfluous. I imagine that, incapable of being haunted, you are incapable of being added to. (*Ibid.*, 606)

Justin's "good night", haunted by the "unthinkable" spectre of death, should have no effect upon Robinson, who does not appear to feel the

[32] The Major's earlier observation of the house – "You might have thought the room had burst into flames" – recalls the apocalyptic fate of the Irish country house in *The Last September* ("SN" 593). Robinson, too, underscores this literary memory, telling Emma, "I know they burnt down the castle [on his demesne] years ago" (*ibid.*, 604).

attack of Queenie-as-memory as Justin does – "you interposed your solidity between me and what might have been the full effects of an exacerbating return" (*ibid.*, 606). And yet importantly, Justin has expressed this sentiment in a letter, a missive that will not reach Robinson until the next day, at least, for the box in which he posts the note "would not be cleared till tomorrow noon" (*ibid.*, 607). Justin's "good night" is thus saved overnight, and again becomes superfluous, its arrival too late to perform. In this way, Justin effects a deliberate negation of the expression, putting the "unthinkable" on hold, unreceived, unthought, until the safety of the day.

Similarly, the Major's repression of Emma's "good night" to her children, telling them at first that she had telephoned to "tell me to tell you to be good", attempts to delay her words, and then at last, to dampen their power, to make them safe or "just": "'What did she say truly?' 'Just good night'" (*ibid.*, 595). "One wants to be able to say 'good night'", Royle argues. "But how? Can one ever truly say 'good night,' in oneself, to oneself or to another, in the name of oneself or of another?"[33] Indeed, the Major's "good night" to his children is always already a repetition of Emma's "good night", haunted – indeed, necessitated – by her absence. When Vivie asks her father, "but suppose she didn't come back?" she demonstrates her awareness of the "unthinkable" present in Emma's "good night", the possibility that she may not return, and that her mother's "good night" may be permanent ("SN" 596).

However, for Vivie, the "anarchy" created by an awareness of mortality even inside the illusion of security inspires life and action (*ibid.*, 597). Recalling her own childhood experience of war, Bowen suggests that "as a child brought up inside the illusion of security, I should have been dinted by the outbreak of war", but that war may have been, "even for children, something of a release".[34] While it is possible to read Vivie's behaviour as an imitation of her mother's desperate flight, attributed to a desire for freedom and for a life beyond the suffocation of her family duties, I want to suggest that her

[33] Royle, *The Uncanny*, 126.
[34] Elizabeth Bowen, "A Year I Remember: 1918" (broadcast 10 March 1949), HRHRC 2.3 (original emphasis).

wild dance is an anarchic assertion of survival and release.[35] For Vivie (unlike her sister, the morbidly named "Di"), the presence of war (the sparring bombers overhead) is vivifying. Now, the children are "born knowing" that security is an illusion, and that every "good night" is haunted by death, and Vivie does not keep it "deadly silent" ("SN" 599). Rather than keeping death in the shadows, Vivie meets its challenge, delighting in the night, and in the chaos and disillusionment of war; in a child's safe way of challenging safety, she refuses the protection of her bed and of her clothes, though she stops short of undoing the locks of the house.[36] "In her skin" ("SN" 596) she runs free around the house, jumps on her mother's bed, and "tattoo[s] her chest, belly and thighs with stars and snakes, red, yellow and blue" (*ibid.*, 597).

It seems that Vivie draws herself as an explosion, imitating not her mother, but the sparks, clouds, and streams of light seen from her window. She at once represents the glory of both life and death, a collapsing admission of both, frolicking in that no-time after "good night" but before sleep. Vivie thus embodies the "new form for thinking and feeling" Justin approaches but fails to act upon:

> For some time we have neither thought nor felt. Our faculties have slowed down without our knowing – they had stopped without our knowing! We know now. Now that there's enough death to challenge being alive we're facing it that, anyhow, we don't live. We're confronted by the impossibility *of* living – unless we can break through to something else. There's been a stop in our senses and in our faculties that's made everything round us so much dead matter – and dead matter we couldn't even displace. We can no longer express ourselves: what we say doesn't even approximate to reality; it only approximates to what's been said .... We've got to break through to the new form – it needs genius. We're precipitated, this moment, between genius and death. I tell you, we must have genius to live at all. (*Ibid.*, 589-90; original emphasis)

[35] This is argued by, for example, Edward Mitchell, "Themes in Elizabeth Bowen's Short Stories", in Bloom, *Elizabeth Bowen*, 49; Shumaker, "Bruised Boys and 'Fallen' Women", 90; and Medoff, "There is No Elsewhere", 75.

[36] "She attempted the front door, but did not dare to touch the chain: she could not get out of the house" ("SN" 596).

In "Summer Night", living "how one can" requires a radical revision of survival; it is Vivie who has the "genius to live at all". Vivie is, like Emma's "good night", mad, haunted, unthinkable. The girl represents "the far side of the nothing" for which Justin strives, beyond "wretched identity" and thus beyond its death, the threatening nothing Aunt Fran fears (*ibid.*, 591). Vivie thus enacts a "break through" – a "new form" in which to live.

Secluded Ireland

"Sunday Afternoon" explores war as an event unimaginable and inexpressible. The war can only be discussed in this environment as "fiction"; it is distanced from reality through its positioning as an adventure story, entertainment for a Sunday afternoon. It is in this emphasis on unthinkability that "Sunday Afternoon" continues to address the concerns of "Summer Night". In this story, the possibility of coherent thinking about the war, or of producing a literature of the events taking place, seems impossible. The story is set in the grounds of a grand Anglo-Irish house in late May, on an "eternalized Sunday afternoon", and describes the teatime visit of Henry Russel, a holidaying Londoner, with his old friends in Ireland. Henry, like Justin, is on "holiday" from war, in what seems to be not only another place, but another time ("SA" 617). He is paraded by his hostess, Mrs Vesey, as a novelty, a storyteller, made to describe and justify the war and his own actions in response to it. His friends treat him almost as a specimen, a typical product of war, before safely packing him off, packing him away, early. Maria, Mrs Vesey's young niece, disturbs the comfort of the afternoon with her confrontations and desire to travel to England, but just as Vivie was protected in "Summer Night", the adults, including Henry, do their best to keep Maria safe, and to discourage her from following him to the glamour of wartime London.

Henry's audience request of him a narration of the trauma of war; from their position of safety, they demand an immediate witness. Henry is encouraged by his friends to tell his story, but the parameters placed upon him – to fit the discourse of war within Mrs Vesey's plea for safety, her request for "nothing dreadful" – make this almost impossible (*ibid.*, 616). Henry thus tells very little, in part because of such difficulties to do with telling, but also because his audience's repeated interruptions to his story demonstrate the difficulty of bridging the gap between danger and safety, between the trauma itself, and its later willed expression. This is the dilemma of the witness: how to express the limit-event in language – can the word "shocking" approach the suffering Henry has observed?[37] As in "Summer Night", the very possibility of thinking and feeling during war, of thinking or feeling "shocked", is called into question: "But as [the bombing] does not connect with the rest of life, it is difficult, you know, to know what one feels", admits Henry: "One's feelings seem to have no language for anything so preposterous. As for thoughts – " ("SA" 617). The bombing, the war, "does not connect with the rest of life" – it is compartmentalized, sheltered, kept safe from consciousness; indeed, for Henry, "the sensations of wartime … locked his inside being". Death, in other words, "does not connect" with, is kept secret from, life, from Henry's determination to survive. In this way, Henry participates in his friends' practice of keeping death "deadly silent", of telling "nothing dreadful", just as they "deny" the "coldness" of the May afternoon, insistently creeping over their bodies (*ibid.*, 616).

For Henry's friends, death is abstract, something that happens to others – "I should see no reason, for instance, why it should happen to me". All they can imagine is the loss of property. Yet for Henry, too, the possibility of annihilation is reduced to "chance": "It was by chance I was out when the place was hit .... But, in fact, I am very glad to remain. To exist." Even though he admits that such destruction "happens to many people", he insists on chance, and emphasizes his survival (*ibid.*, 619). Yet "Sunday Afternoon" may be read as a figuration of Henry's changing "attitude towards death",[38] for by the story's end Henry recognizes his return to London as a return to "the zone of death". His desire to protect Maria from the threat of death forces him to acknowledge its presence, and his longing for the past becomes a longing for naivety ("SA" 621).[39] Until this moment, Maria's "whole existence has been in contradistinction" – indeed, so

---

[37] "'Are things there as shocking as they say – are or they more shocking?' … Henry, in fact, was just beginning to twiddle this far-off word 'shocking' round in his mind" ("SA" 617). The inadequacy of the word "shocking" is also suggested in "A Love Story" (504).

[38] Freud, "Timely Reflections on War and Death", 185.

[39] Henry wishes to protect Maria from her belief that travel to London will be a kind of "dying into life", as Harold Bloom puts it ("Introduction" to Bloom, *Elizabeth Bowen*, 3).

has his own ("SA" 622). Now he realizes, as Freud states, that "People are really dying, not individually now, but in large numbers, often tens of thousands in a single day. And it is no longer a matter of chance .... accumulation abolishes chance."[40]

For Bowen, it was the end of the war, the removal of a perpetual reminder of one's own mortality that stopped her short. She recalls:

> I was terrified by the vacuum, the absolute full-stop, in my thoughts, in my being, in my soul. It seemed to me, suddenly, that I had grown up without having the capacity to feel.[41]

Her words echo Henry's, for where language should be, there is only a terrifying "vacuum" – nothing. Here exists a double-bind, for while the trauma of war and of death is itself unthinkable, without it, thought stops. War is the only thought, and yet the thought that cannot be expressed. "The simple way to put it was", Bowen later wrote:

> "One cannot take things in." What was happening was out of all proportion to our faculties for knowing, thinking and checking up.[42]

Thus in "Sunday Afternoon", Ronald Cuffe announces the impossibility of a literature of war:

> "About what is important," announced Maria, "it seems that no one can tell one anything. There is really nothing, till one knows it oneself."
>
> "Henry is probably right," said Ronald Cuffe, "in considering that this – this outrage is *not* important. There is no place for it in human experience; it apparently cannot make a place of its own. It will have no literature."
>
> "Literature!" said Maria. "One can see, Mr Cuffe, that *you* have always been safe!" ("SA" 618; original emphasis)

To even think of literature, Maria's expostulation suggests, signifies safety, for creative production can only ever belong to a higher order of a hierarchy of needs. Yet, more than this, Ronald's statement

---

[40] Freud, "Timely Reflections on War and Death", 185.

[41] Bowen, "A Year I Remember", 18.

[42] Bowen, "Postscript to *The Demon Lover*", 96.

proposes that a place should not be kept for the war, as Maria keeps a place for Henry at the table, and that such an experience should not be preserved, for language cannot approach it (*ibid.*, 619). Second-hand thought, literary testimony, is impossible, "there is really nothing, till one knows it oneself". The paradox is that Ronald and Maria are themselves fictional products of the literature of wartime, so that "Sunday Afternoon" defies the claim that war trauma cannot be represented but also, as Richard Greaves has noted of wartime short fiction in general, that "There is, perhaps, something paradoxical in the idea that the short story can provide a form for responses to such epic events as World Wars I and II".[43] Henry's stops and starts, his stuttering attempt to express his life, his ambiguities, his silences, are those of the narrative. Perhaps, this text suggests, this is what literature of war, of trauma, could look like (it would, for Bowen, reach its fullest expression in her wartime novel, *The Heat of the Day*). Stories of a disintegrated life are, like the life itself, the destroyed wartime landscape, and an insufficient language, filled with gaps. Survival of such an experience, the necessity of keeping a place for it, thus required new forms of thinking and writing trauma.

Fantastic Ireland

Survival is life's resistance against death. For Bowen, wartime survival seems to have been a collective effort: the accumulation of lives – real lives, fictional lives – shored up against "the annihilation that was threatening it", the accumulation of people dying.[44] Indeed, Freud points out that literature itself can be a site of "compensation" for what I read as a Bowenesque "meaner living":

> So we have no option but to find compensations in the world of fiction, in literature, in the theatre for that which we have lost in life .... In the sphere of fiction we find the plurality of lives that we need. We die in our identification with one hero, but survive him and are ready to die a second time, equally unarmed, with another.[45]

---

[43] Richard Greaves, "Responses to War: 1914-18 and 1939-45", in *A Companion to the British and Irish Short Story*, eds Cheryl Alexander Malcolm and David Malcolm, Chichester: Wiley-Blackwell, 2008, 35.

[44] Bowen, "Postscript to *The Demon Lover*", 97.

[45] Freud, "Timely Reflections on War and Death", 185.

Fiction and fantasy, "often childishly innocent", are "compensations" for death and destruction, and one means of consolation during wartime.[46] For example, in "Mysterious Kôr" (1944), the high-tide mark of hallucination in *The Demon Lover*, Pepita and her soldier lover, Arthur, wander the dead city streets, playing out their fantasy of the ghostly Kôr, the mystical city of Rider Haggard's novel, *She* (1886).[47] In a way similar to Queenie's projection of the blissful past onto the threatening present, Pepita reconstructs blitzed London as the fictional city of her reading childhood, thereby casting it in the safety and security of that period. Pepita and Arthur inhabit the fantasy – what John Bayley terms "her comfort, her safe place" – and maintain the illusion of survival through their plans for procreation ("MK" 731).[48]

In her post-war essay, "Out of a Book", Bowen addresses this interaction between life and fiction:

> For the child, any real-life scene that has once been sucked into the ambiance of the story is affected, or infected, forever ... Such a thing, place or scene cannot again be walked past indifferently; it exerts a pull and sets up a tremor; and it is to indent the memory for life.[49]

The fluidity of this relationship describes the hallucinatory or supernatural aspects of Bowen's writing, especially her wartime short stories, which often arise from a consideration of what Petra Rau calls "the fictitiousness of (wartime) reality".[50] What Bowen terms the

---

[46] "Dreams by night, and the fantasies – these often childishly innocent – with which formerly matter-of-fact people consoled themselves by day were compensations" (Bowen, "Postscript to *The Demon Lover*", 96).

[47] "Mysterious Kôr" is the final story in *The Demon Lover*, the collection in which, Bowen notes, she found "a rising tide of hallucination" (*ibid.*, 96).

[48] John Bayley, *The Short Story: Henry James to Elizabeth Bowen*, Brighton: Harvester, 1988, 169.

[49] Elizabeth Bowen, "Out of a Book" (1946), in *The Mulberry Tree*, 52.

[50] Petra Rau, "The Common Frontier: Fictions of Alterity in Elizabeth Bowen's *The Heat of the Day* and Graham Greene's *The Ministry of Fear*", *Literature and History*, XIV/1 (May 2005), 32. Keri Walsh suggests that "Stories of the London Blitz, including 'The Happy Autumn Fields' and 'Mysterious Kôr', are best understood as deriving their haunting effects from Bowen's merging of surrealist techniques with an Anglo-Irish Gothic tradition" ("Elizabeth Bowen, Surrealist", *Eire-Ireland*, XLII/3-4 [Fall/Winter 2007], 129).

"overlapping and haunting of life by fiction", begins in childhood.[51] Here, as in wartime, fiction compensates for the "insufficiency", or impoverishment, "of so-called real life" – it fleshes out the "otherwise constricted" life.[52] Children read sensationally, "unthinkingly", she observes, but when such children grow up, "it becomes an enormity, inside the full-sized body, to read without the brain".[53] Reading "without the brain" is to read with the body, sensuously, and on face-value – to remain innocent of reality. To read "without the brain" is to seek consolation in fantasy, to read without knowledge, without thought, to throw oneself entirely into the world of fiction and of life outside death; in wartime, it is to leave behind the traumatic present and the recognition of death.

In that essay, Bowen is concerned, in particular, with the ways in which people console themselves with literature of the past: "*Reading is* an aid", she notes, "and the past, lately, has proved one unfailing source – memoirs, biography, old diaries found in old desks, agreeable works of history, rich historical novels".[54] Memory in, for example, "The Happy Autumn Fields", is a site of safety.[55] Positioning the self within a psychic space preserved for safekeeping, and moreover, within a temporal space which must remain untouched by war, becomes a coping mechanism in Bowen's wartime short fiction. That is, in these stories memory becomes an escape from the present, and thereby a refusal of the possibility of death. Caruth's argument that the cause of trauma "is a shock that appears to work very much like a bodily threat but is in fact a break in the mind's experience of time", here suggests that trauma occurs when "a bodily threat" overcomes psychic refuge in the past, collapsing the temporal boundaries constructed to preclude death, and thus annihilating the self "in the mind's experience of time".[56]

These temporal constructions founded in the reading of old documents – "a musty old leather box gaping open with God knows

---

[51] Bowen, "Out of a Book", 48.
[52] *Ibid.*, 49, 51.
[53] *Ibid.*, 48, 50.
[54] Bowen, "The Cult of Nostalgia" (broadcast 4 August 1951), HRHRC 2.3 (original emphasis).
[55] Ellmann notes that "The Happy Autumn Fields" "explores these compensatory dreams of plenitude" (*The Shadow Across the Page*, 169).
[56] Caruth, *Unclaimed Experience*, 61.

what – junk, illegible letters, diaries, yellow photographs, chiefly plaster and dust" – instigate the hallucinatory action of "The Happy Autumn Fields", a fragmented narrative which juxtaposes Mary, in the dangerous present of London in the Blitz, with her idyllic "dream" of Sarah, in Victorian Ireland.[57] Like Queenie in "Summer Night", Mary seeks refuge in the past. The story opens on Sarah and her family walking in the fields; abruptly, Mary, and the reader, are removed from this scene as she awakens from that dream with a cry. After Mary's lover, Travis, urges her to leave the house, which is in danger of collapsing around her, she again falls asleep and returns to her life as Sarah, who has the hallucinatory awareness that she has been absent for some time. The story concludes when Mary awakens again, devastated that her survival of yet another bomb has precluded the possibility of her return: "The one way back to the fields was barred by Mary's surviving the fall of ceiling" ("HAF" 683). Yet, it is also possible that her survival has been enabled by the processes of her dream: Mary has "partaken of [her] fiction's body".[58]

Caruth has identified this preoccupation with survival, with life rather than death, in Freud's writing on wartime trauma in, for example, *Beyond the Pleasure Principle* and *Moses and Monotheism*. "*What does it mean to survive?*" she asks, for "It is only by recognizing traumatic experience as a paradoxical relation between destructiveness and survival that we can also recognize the legacy of incomprehensibility at the heart of catastrophic experience".[59] This incomprehensibility, I suggest, is the "unthinkable" inherent in Emma's "good night" and in Henry's unspoken thought. Indeed, this lacunae "between destructiveness and survival" may also be seen to represent Freud's "deadly silen[ce]", the impossibility of thinking one's own death. It is this very gap in thought which, Freud states, war forces one to confront, for in order to think one's own survival, one

[57] Elizabeth Bowen, "The Happy Autumn Fields" (1944), in *Collected Stories*, 677. Hereafter cited parenthetically as "HAF". Lee points out that "There are Victorian diary entries in *Bowen's Court* which inspired 'The Happy Autumn Fields'" (*Elizabeth Bowen*, 18).

[58] Bowen, "Out of a Book", 52.

[59] Caruth, *Unclaimed Experience*, 58, 60 (original emphasis). *Beyond the Pleasure Principle* and *Moses and Monotheism*, Caruth suggests, "represent Freud's formulation of trauma as a theory of the peculiar incomprehensibility of human survival" (*ibid.*, 58).

has also to admit the possibility of death. Safety, it seems, can only exist in relation to an awareness of danger.

"The Happy Autumn Fields" figures this admission as Mary's dream enacts a repeated attempt to be aware of the threat of death. Mary's dream is an unconscious confrontation of the possibility of her death that will permit her survival. Caruth states:

> The return of the traumatic experience in the dream is not the signal of the direct experience but, rather, of the attempt to overcome the fact that it was *not* direct, to attempt to master what was never fully grasped in the first place. Not having truly known the threat of death in the past, the survivor is forced, continually, to confront it over and over again. For consciousness then, the act of survival, as the experience of trauma, is the repeated confrontation with the necessity and impossibility of grasping the threat to one's own life.[60]

While Mary, in her dream as Sarah, admits to "the feeling of dislocation, the formless dread", she "never fully grasp[s]", she never comprehends, to what this "dread" is attributed ("HAF" 681). In the hallucinatory repetitions of this necessary and yet impossible acknowledgement of Eugene's traumatic death, Mary's psyche seeks to save her life, to make possible her survival in the threatening present, in a manner which echoes the behaviour of Portia in *The Death of the Heart*: "Your own nerves know that [the house is not safe], even if you don't: … Your will keeps driving your self, but it can't be driven the whole way – it makes its own get-out: sleep." (*Ibid.*, 676)

Mary is what Corcoran terms "an unexpected survivor";[61] her awakening to the shock of her own survival occurs only when Sarah has come to recognize the threat of death made against Eugene, as Henrietta implores her to reiterate her promise that "Whatever tries to come between me and Sarah becomes nothing" ("HAF" 683). And Sarah's silence – "Sarah, who, as once before, could not speak" – the interrupted thought on which the Victorian narrative is disrupted and

---

[60] *Ibid.*, 62 (original emphasis).

[61] Corcoran, *The Enforced Return*, 148. "The trauma of the nightmare does not simply consist in the experience *within* the dream, but in *the experience of waking from it* …. It is not only the dream that surprises consciousness but, indeed, the very *waking itself* that constitutes the surprise" (Caruth, *Unclaimed Experience*, 64; original emphasis).

returns to the present, figures the "unthinkable", her awareness of the threat of annihilation, and thus enables Mary's awareness of the necessity of survival. Although Mary laments the "cruel[ty]" of her dream, it has achieved its purpose, for "now how am I to help laying that like a pattern against the poor stuff of everything else?" (*Ibid.*, 684) Although she can no longer remain in the blissful naivety of immortality, any more than she could remain in the idyll of the Irish countryside with her dear sister, Henrietta, this relinquishment enables her survival in the present.

"We are still alive"

Bowen's wartime short fiction is a literature of survival, and dependent on Irish space for this to happen. Each story refuses or overcomes annihilation, consistently privileging life over death, the safety of the psyche over the danger posed to the body. These stories determine an optimism necessary for survival in a war-torn present, an ideology of safety that resists destruction. What is kept safe throughout these stories, the thought preserved, is succinctly expressed in "London, 1940": "It is a fine morning and we are still alive."[62]

[62] Bowen, "London, 1940", 23.

CHAPTER 6

UNKNOWN: *THE HEAT OF THE DAY*

> To know what I knew, to keep my knowing unknown, unknown all the time to be acting on it – I tell you, everything fell into place round me. (*HD* 307)

> A frightful mystery, a secret to make you tremble .... A secret always makes you tremble. Not simply quiver or shiver, which also happens sometimes, but tremble .... One doesn't know *why one trembles*. This limit to knowledge no longer only relates to the cause or unknown event, the unseen or unknown that makes us tremble .... Why does the irrepressible take this form?[1]

Bowen's novel of wartime London, *The Heat of the Day*, constructs the unknown and the effect of the unknown. Although this is a text which has been described as Bowen's "spy novel", *The Heat of the Day* does not expose, but rather perpetuates the traumatic unknown.[2] In this chapter I will explore the way in which Bowen's novel of wartime London textualizes the Modernist "shock of the new" – the literal shakes and shocks that describe the effect of trauma: that is, it figures in form and in content the Derridean "unseen or unknown that makes us tremble", as well as the trembling itself. I will demonstrate how *The Heat of the Day* works as a trembling narrative of the modern world: refusing the silence or unspeakability of the "typical" writing of trauma, Bowen's novel writes the uncertainty of wartime, and a broader terror of the unknown which characterizes the first half of the twentieth century (and arguably, since then). More specifically,

---

[1] Jacques Derrida, *The Gift of Death*, trans. David Wills, Chicago, IL: University of Chicago Press, 1995, 53-55 (original emphasis).

[2] See, for example, Corcoran, *The Enforced Return*, 187; Patrick Deer, *Culture in Camouflage: War, Empire, and Modern British Literature*, Oxford: Oxford University Press, 2009, 184; and in detail, Allan Hepburn, *Intrigue: Espionage and Culture*, New Haven, CT: Yale University Press, 2005, 134-65.

it does this by exploring the secrecy of wartime and of wartime work, and of romantic relationships; the unknown dead, and the fear of an unknown or unrecognizable self; and above all, the unknown trauma which "makes us tremble".

I see Bowen's modernity to lie in her response to the condition of anxiety and trauma; like other Modernist writers such as Virginia Woolf, Rosamond Lehmann and Jean Rhys, Bowen adopts this new literary form to try to evoke its disturbances of ordered space and time. Indeed, Modernist fiction, with its emphasis on psychological representation, is particularly well suited to narrativize the memory of trauma, which in its broadest terms, is nonlinear and scarred by silences. As Caruth points out, it is the very belatedness of its experience which characterizes the traumatic event. She recognizes that "trauma is not locatable in the simple violent or original event in an individual's past, but rather in the way that its very unassimilated nature – the way it was precisely not known in the first instance – returns to haunt the survivor later on".[3] LaCapra takes this even further, and suggests that we might read Modernism itself as post-traumatic. He argues that Woolf's work, for example, "is in no sense a conventional narrative but one that both traces the effects of trauma and somehow, at least linguistically, tries to come to terms with those effects, so that they will be inscribed and recalled but perhaps reconfigured in ways that make them not entirely disabling".[4]

But Bowen's work differs from that of her contemporaries in its concern for the ways in which writing survives trauma and works towards its ethical representation. Bowen's wartime novel is a particularly interesting example because it is here that she records the traumatic effects of war in language and thereby enacts the permutations of the wartime known and unknown in a commemoration of the physical and the psychological state of Second World War London. Precisely because of the "interruptions" of its "subject", Bowen later wrote, the novel was not completed until some years after the end of the Second World War: "[*The Heat of the Day* took] longer to write than any other of my novels; partly because it was a good deal interrupted by what is in the main its subject, the war,

---

[3] Caruth, *Unclaimed Experience*, 4.
[4] LaCapra, *History and Memory*, 168.

and partly because so many psychological as well as technical difficulties kept cropping up in the course of it."[5]

The Heat of the Day records these "psychological" and "technical difficulties" in a demonstration of the trembling continuation of, or aftershock from, the traumatic event of war. And when Robert Kelway finally reveals his espionage activities to be in part a consequence of his traumatic retreat in the First World War (as part of that "army of freedom queueing up to be taken off by pleasure boats" [*HD* 306]), the novel's events are shown as always already a continuation of the effects of the earlier conflict. Indeed, we might say this is true of all Bowen's work: her entire *oeuvre* could be read as a quaking post-traumatic event or effect. In all of Bowen's writing trembles the shimmering "heat of the day before" (*WL* 9).

The Heat of the Day engages with these as literary effects; in other words, the novel performs a literature of modern trauma (and specifically, a literature of war). This is most clearly signified by the narrative's complicated sentence structures, which constitute a kind of a trembling or stammering, a syntactical disruption which may be read as a continuing traumatic effect or, indeed, symptom. The "queer" order of words in *The Heat of the Day*, "the jars, 'jingles' and awkwardnesses" work, Bowen wrote in a letter to her publisher, to make a "psychological impact" – to have an effect upon the reader.[6] She was, she later said, "trying to put language to what for me was a totally new use, and what, perhaps was, showed itself to be a quite impossible use".[7] But I want to take Bowen to task in her assertion of the "impossible use" of language to represent trauma. Language, in post-war *The Heat of the Day*, has undergone a seismic upset as a result of an event that has already occurred. In this sense, the novel's very form is always and everywhere constituted as symptomatic of the war's ongoing traumatic, tremulous effects; moreover, and perhaps more powerfully, this continuation of an unknown trembling may also be seen as an anticipation of further or repeated trauma, as an effect of repression and anxiety.

I agree, then, with Lee's assertion that this novel is an example of "strain[ed]" writing, but I suggest that more than this, what is so

[5] Elizabeth Bowen, "Material for the *Broadsheet*" (n.d.), HRHRC 1.5, 1.
[6] Elizabeth Bowen, letter to Daniel George (2 June 1948), HRHRC 10.4, 1-2.
[7] Bowen, "Elizabeth Bowen and Jocelyn Brooke in Conversation", 12.

interesting about *The Heat of the Day* is that it is an example of writing that trembles in reaction and in apprehension.[8] As Derrida points out:

> … trembling, at least as a signal or symptom, is something that has already taken place, as in the case of an earthquake [*tremblement de terre*] or when one trembles all over. It is no longer preliminary even if, unsettling everything so as to imprint upon the body an irrepressible shaking, the event that makes one tremble portends and threatens still. It suggests that violence is going to break out again, that some traumatism will insist on being repeated.[9]

Derrida's earthquake as a metaphor for the repetition of trauma takes on further significance in the novel's context of the Blitz on London during 1940 and 1941, for those fifty-seven consecutive nights of bombing had sociological, physiological, psychological and narratological implications and reverberations, and constituted a "general rocking of London and one's own mind" (*HD* 98). Bennett and Royle have described *The Heat of the Day* as an example of "blitz-writing".[10] I want to suggest that the tremulous narrative might also be portrayed, in Bowen's own terms, as an "earthquake stor[y]" (*HD* 69), a text that is an effect of, or set in shuddering motion by, a city at war.

The narrative opens, like Bowen's previous novel, *The Death of the Heart*, in Regent's Park, although its atmosphere, over a decade later (specifically, "the first Sunday of September 1942" [*ibid.*, 4]), is vastly changed; indeed, as Lee notes, to compare these scenes in the two novels which, in the corpus of Bowen's work, bracket the Second World War, is to have a "vivid sense of what the war did to this part of London".[11] Shattering and fragmentation has, in *The Heat of the Day*, spread beyond the icy pond of *The Death of the Heart*; Bowen notes of the "apparent disjection between the characters and the scenes" in the later novel that she "was aiming to give an effect of fortuity, of a smashed up pattern with its fragments invecting on one

---

[8] Lee, *Elizabeth Bowen*, 158.
[9] Derrida, *Gift of Death*, 53-54 (translator's emphasis).
[10] Bennett and Royle, *Elizabeth Bowen and the Dissolution of the Novel*, 94.
[11] Lee, *Elizabeth Bowen*, 107.

another, drifting and tapping rather like the broken ice which is described in the opening passage [of *The Death of the Heart*]".[12]

The introductory scene is one of only two in which both strands of the novel's plot intersect (the other occurs when Harrison and Stella unexpectedly meet Louie in a café): Louie Lewis, "a woman of about twenty-seven, with the roughened hair and still slightly upward expression of someone who has been lying flat on the grass", is part of a crowd of "shabby Londoners" and "exiled foreigners" listening to a Viennese orchestra in the park's open-air theatre (*HD* 7). Her appearance is catalogued in professional detail by her neighbour in the audience, the counterspy Harrison, a man whose face has "a gate behind it" (*ibid.*, 9). Harrison forms the hinge of the novel's doubled plot, the parallel stories of Louie Lewis and of Stella Rodney. After the concert, Harrison arrives at Stella's London flat to tell her the information on which the narrative turns: that her lover, Robert, is passing secret information to the enemy, an act that has, he tells her, "For a good bit of time … been suspected; now it's established, known" (*ibid.*, 35). However, if Stella becomes his lover, Harrison slyly states, he will refrain from reporting Robert to his superiors. The novel's suspense, then, as Renée C. Hoogland has noted, derives not from its plot but rather from its psychology – from the Modernist innovations in character.[13] Stella responds to Harrison's revelation neither one way nor the other, but suspicion of Robert has been implanted: she does not tell her lover of Harrison's visit, and begins to watch him herself, noting his habits and behaviour, and suggesting a visit to his family home, Holme Dene, to look, as Harrison puts it, "at the first place where rot could start" (*HD* 144). "You succeed in making a spy of me", Stella observes (*ibid.*, 152). Eventually she confronts Robert and, after some time, during a lengthy discussion at Stella's flat (much of the novel is constructed of evasive and non-committal dialogue), he confesses. Convinced that he is being watched and will be arrested if he is seen leaving her home, Robert escapes through a skylight, only to "fall or leap from the roof" to his death (*ibid.*, 327).

---

[12] Bowen, "Elizabeth Bowen and Jocelyn Brooke in Conversation", 1.

[13] Renée C. Hoogland, *Elizabeth Bowen: A Reputation in Writing*, New York: New York University Press, 1994, 119.

Running parallel to Stella's plot is that of her working-class counterpart Louie, left alone in London after her parents are killed by a bomb, and her husband, Tom, is called up. Yet even while Louie's construction of a female community with Connie, an ARP warden, works to evoke the mythical sense of comradeship in London during the Blitz, she remains lonely and promiscuous. By the novel's conclusion Louie has given birth to an illegitimate son she names Thomas Victor, in a strange concatenation of the name of her own husband, and of Stella's. The novel closes on this child born of an unknown father, and on whom devolves the signification of the narrative's two unknown men. Although most critics read this conclusion as hopeful or as symbolic of survival, I want rather to think about this image of the infant, held high by his mother in the hope that "he too might see, and perhaps remember", as a permutation of Bowen's typical "threshold" conclusion (*ibid.*, 372).[14] In this context, the physically and genealogically suspended child, vessel of the unknown dead may, like the novel itself, be read as a traumatic effect, and as a signification of the continuation of trembling into the "thoughtless" future (*HD* 372).

Textual effects

Such trembling, quaking, rippling effects are also at work in the novel's opening scene in Regent's Park. The "disturbing" (*ibid.*, 3) music played by musicians with "the faces and hands of ghosts" (*ibid.*, 11) draws into its shadowy epicentre, "by the sensation that they were missing something" (*ibid.*, 3), the "solitary" strangers of the urban warzone; they are, in turn, pursued by "those who had followed the others into the theatre automatically" in a chain of unknown

[14] See, for example, Jordan, *How Will the Heart Endure*, 168; Lee, *Elizabeth Bowen*, 175; Barbara Bellow Watson, "Variations on an Enigma: Elizabeth Bowen's War Novel", in Bloom, *Elizabeth Bowen*, 83; Damon Marcel DeCoste, "The Literary Response to the Second World War", in *A Companion to the British and Irish Novel, 1945-2000*, ed. Brian W. Shaffer, Malden, MA: Blackwell, 2005, 16; and Karen Schneider, *Loving Arms: British Women Writing the Second World War*, Lexington: University Press of Kentucky, 1997, 98. Brook Miller, on the other hand, argues that Bowen does not leave Louie "as a liberated figure for hope, but as a subject desperately striving to maintain her own fictions by crafting an identity for her son that represses the fact of his paternity" ("Narrative, Meaning and Agency in *The Heat of the Day*", in Osborn, *New Critical Perspectives*, 146).

consequence (*ibid.*, 5). In the orchestra's pauses are tremulous outbreaks: the musicians "turn over their sheets of music" (*ibid.*, 7), the audience bestows a "ripple of clapping" (*ibid.*, 6), Louie's programme "fluttered to the ground" (*ibid.*, 10). But this rippling and fluttering is a continuation of the "already … drifting" leaves which, in the novel's opening paragraph, turn over, like the sheet-music, "crepitating as though in the act of dying" (*ibid.*, 3). In turn, the narrative itself has been set in motion by an event unstated at this point (the novel delays temporal specification of wartime for two pages), but which has already occurred outside the narrative frame. This is a season, the narrator states, which had never "been more felt" (*ibid.*, 98). The rippling atmosphere of the novel's first scene describes, to use Derrida's words "a signal or symptom" of "something that has already taken place", and that "will insist on being repeated".[15] Everything quivers, anxiously, vibrating on the threshold of the "last silent crackle of sunset" (*HD* 7), in echo of those "crepitating" leaves, suspended in "the act of dying" (*ibid.*, 3), like the concert-goers who "paused in the gateways doubtfully – all they had left behind was in sunshine, while this hollow which was the source of music was found to be also the source of dusk" (*ibid.*, 7).

"War", states Bowen in *Bowen's Court*, "is not an accident: it is an outcome. One cannot look back too far to ask, of what?" (*BC* 454) And in *The Heat of the Day*, Harrison observes that, "War, if you come to think of it, hasn't started anything that wasn't there already" (*HD* 33). A narrative of personal and (inter)national "outcome", *The Heat of the Day* positions war as an effect, a tremor of unknown origin. Even while the novel provokes this backward look towards the unknown or secret event, its consequences ripple on towards the inevitability of darkness and death, the "incoming tide" of evening (*ibid.*, 4). Those quivering leaves do, after all, continue to fall like bombs (and like Robert) throughout the novel, in an autumnal resignation to temporal continuity, as Stella recognizes when she travels to her son's inherited property in Ireland, Mount Morris: "The seeming of this to be forever was astonishing – until a leaf fell slowly, veering towards her eyes as though she had brought time with her into the wood" (*ibid.*, 197). This is a leaf already "plucked still quivering" by the ancestral ladies Stella imagines to have "gone not quite mad" at

---

[15] Derrida, *Gift of Death*, 53-54.

Mount Morris; one of the leaves to the sound of "crisping" piles of which she first came to know Robert (*ibid.*, 100). And if *The Heat of the Day* is felt as an effect of a precipitating tremor, it might also be said that these September falling leaves continue those which fall in Bowen's earlier novel of civil unrest, *The Last September*. In both novels, melancholic autumn is the temporal setting for social collapse.

Trauma, war, in *The Heat of the Day*, is then partly an effect, and partly produces effects, so that it is affecting, and infecting, "malarial" (*ibid.*, 100):

> You did not know what you might not be tuning in to, you could not say what you might not be picking up – affected, infected you were at every turn. Receiver, conductor, carrier – which was Louie, what was she doomed to be? (*Ibid.*, 278)

No originating point of infection can be identified, and Louie's own role in the chain of effect is similarly unknown. Bowen also uses this metaphor of infection – picking up, perhaps, on this sense of war as a theatre for the "act of dying" – in her secret reports on Eire, prepared for the Ministry of Information as part of her "espionage" work during the war: "I believe that with many people [in Eire] there is a nebulous feeling that war is *infectious*: the more belligerents accumulate in the Six Counties, the more likely it is that the 'germ' will spread", she wrote: "War, in fact, is not *entered* but 'caught' – or picked up – just as, passively and unwillingly, one catches or picks up measles."[16] War, then, is a sweeping wave of a peculiarly modern infection, an effect of unknown germination.

Sexual effects

Stella and Robert's romantic relationship is also a traumatic effect, a trembling, set in motion by an unidentifiable or unknown introduction. Their first words to one another are lost in the quaking noise of a bomb:

[16] Elizabeth Bowen (as Elizabeth Cameron), "Notes on Eire", The National Archives, DO130/28, 9 February 1942 (original emphasis).

> She returned to Robert – both having caught a breath, they fixed their eyes expectantly on each other's lips. Both waited, both spoke at once, unheard ….
>
> Now down a shaft of anticipating silence the bomb swung whistling. With the shock of detonation, still to be heard, four walls of in here yawped in then bellied out; bottles danced on glass; a distortion ran through the view. The detonation dulled off into the cataracting roar of a split building: direct hit, somewhere else.
>
> It was the demolition of an entire moment: he and she stood at attention till the glissade stopped. What they *had* both been saying, or been on the point of saying, neither of them ever now were to know. Most first words have the nature of being trifling; theirs from having been lost began to have the significance of a lost clue. What they next said, what they said instead, they forgot: there are questions which if not asked at the start are not asked later; so those they never did ask …. The extraordinary battle in the sky transfixed them; they might have stayed forever on the eve of being in love. (*HD* 104-105; original emphasis)

Like the novel's opening scenes, then, Stella and Robert's romantic relationship is suspended, "transfixed" in anticipation. These moments of trembling are traumatic effects of modern collisions of stillness and movement, "distortion[s]" exemplified by that strange figuration of immobility and reverberation, the "shock-stopped" clock on the wall of the restaurant in which Stella and Robert dine, as well as by their two unsynchronized watches (*ibid.*, 107). Their simultaneously "unheard" words are not only drowned out, but replaced by an explosion, so that their "being in love" – and the narrative itself – is a form of shrapnel, traumatic issue of this bomb, and of the war. Stella and Robert's relationship is not only "premised on a stranger's death", as Allan Hepburn asserts; perhaps more disturbingly, it is a consequence of a temporal death, the "demolition" of their first moment.[17] And while Hepburn persuasively argues that the couple's "sense of timelessness, a symptom of trauma brought on by bombardment and accentuated by pervasive darkness, is a symptom of being scared to death", I want to suggest that their romantic relationship is a traumatic effect or "symptom" of the "timelessness"

[17] Hepburn, *Intrigue: Espionage and Culture*, 146.

wrought by the bomb.[18] Stella and Robert are "an accident", they "*are* friends of circumstance – war, this isolation, this atmosphere in which everything goes on and nothing's said" (*HD* 210; original emphasis). The lost first words of their romance shape their relationship around this secret, this irrecoverable "lost clue". If it is true, as Cixous asserts, that "The true secret causes the most suffering, because it is the exact figure of death", and that "If we have a secret we don't tell then we truly are a tomb", then Stella and Robert's romance is structured, from the outset, by a figuration of death.[19] Together they mourn their temporal and linguistic loss – the "apprehension" of which Stella later awakes to (*HD* 105); they are united ("kindred spirits" [*ibid.*, 104]) in their shared grief for a dead or absent moment, and for secret words which, once "trifling", take on the (traumatic) "significance of a lost clue" (*ibid.*, 104).

The effect of time is the binding element of Stella and Robert's romance; but so too, it distorts the traditional dyad:

> Their time sat in the third place at their table .... The relation of people to one another is subject to the relation of each to time, to what is happening. If this has not been always felt – and as to that who is to know? – it has begun to be felt, irrevocably. On from now, every moment, with more and more of what had been "now" behind it, would be going on adding itself to the larger story. (*Ibid.*, 217)

Time is the third presence in their relationship. Political and social trauma, in this novel, works pervasively, destabilizing, distorting, trembling the traditional dyadic conception of romantic love. But note the way in which temporal unknownness intrudes upon, and becomes a part of, the effect (just as it intrudes upon the relationship). It is not just time, then, but its unknownness, which takes the third place. And it is the unknown, which has, as I have argued, set in trembling motion Stella and Robert's romance, and which now comes to describe their affair.

This is the traumatic void with which the unknown Harrison, "love's necessary missing part", is aligned, and within which he

---

[18] *Ibid.*, 148.

[19] Hélène Cixous, *Three Steps on the Ladder of Writing*, trans. Sarah Cornell and Susan Sellers, New York: Columbia University Press, 1993, 42.

appears (*ibid*., 361). Harrison is unrecognizable, unidentifiable, and more than that, nullified: he is, at Cousin Francis' funeral, "not known to be anyone" (*ibid*., 77), while Louie, early on, tells the counterspy, "I don't know you … I don't even know who you are" (*ibid*., 10), and Robert, too, asks, "is he anybody?" (*ibid*., 223). Even Harrison's Christian name – which is also Robert – remains unknown until his final meeting with Stella. It is his figuration as a traumatizing or disruptive element and moreover, as unknown, as nobody from nowhere, which aligns Harrison with the absent or dead moment that functions as the beginning of Stella and Robert's romantic relationship. By stepping into the space of temporal death, the space opened up by the explosion, Harrison – who, like a time bomb, enters Stella's life "on the quiver of the appointed hour as though attached to the very works of the clock" (*ibid*., 21) and is, moreover, able to anticipate the explosive vibrations of her telephone (*ibid*., 45) – works in a similar way: he distorts or trembles the romantic dyad and is able to wreak consequence. Robert's "rival" (*ibid*., 209) for Stella's love, Harrison impregnates her with the doubt that his third presence signifies: "the story takes – seeds itself in some crack" (*ibid*., 212). And just as Harrison anticipates the ringing of a telephone, he also makes Stella expectant of disaster:

> In the night, how did I not hear it ticking under the pillow like your watch? …. We have not, then, been really alone together for the last two months. You're two months gone with this. (*Ibid*., 213)

Harrison and his "seed", his "story", distends the romantic dyad; it represents a traumatically modern distortion of Stella and Robert's "continuous narrative of love" (*ibid*., 108) and recasts Stella as the "*femme fatale*" (*ibid*., 89). Blameless, in her divorce as now, Stella is nonetheless positioned by Robert and by Harrison as the focus of suspicion, as espionage is reinscribed through "sexual perversion and moral corruption" – problems associated with women and with the female body.[20]

Inculcated as part of Stella and Robert's unity is their desire to avoid being as irrevocably unknown as their first words, to escape the

[20] Tammy M. Proctor, *Female Intelligence: Women and Espionage in the First World War*, New York: New York University Press, 2003, 2.

terrible fate of anonymity suffered by London's "unknown dead" (*HD* 99). It is for this reason that Louie, who is part of the ghostly unknown living, "of meaning only to an absent person" (*ibid.*, 161-62), seeks sites of belonging, and forms attachments – socially and sexually – to "unknown people" (*ibid.*, 13). Her obsession with reading newspapers, for example, is a function of her desire to be known, for what she finds in the newspaper is "an address to or else account of herself" (*ibid.*, 168). Her conversation with Harrison at the concert which opens the novel is a means of "forc[ing] him to notice her", to momentarily cease to be unknown: "her object was to feel that she, Louie, *was*" (*ibid.*, 12; original emphasis).

> Most of all the dead, from mortuaries, from under cataracts of rubble, made their anonymous presence – not as today's dead but as yesterday's living – felt through London. Uncounted, they continued to move in shoals through the city day, pervading everything to be seen or heard or felt with their torn-off senses, drawing on this tomorrow they had expected – for death cannot be so sudden as all that. Absent from the routine which had been life, they stamped upon that routine their absence – not knowing who the dead were, you could not know which might be the staircase somebody for the first time was not mounting this morning, or at which street corner the newsvendor missed a face, or which trains and buses in the homegoing rush were this evening lighter by at least one passenger.
>
> These unknown dead reproached those left living not by their death, which might any night be shared, but by their unknownness, which could not be mended now. Who had the right to mourn them, not having cared that they had lived? (*Ibid.*, 99)

Death, too, is "felt" as an effect in the wartime scene of *The Heat of the Day*; it is a trembling continuation, the inertia towards an "expected" "tomorrow", of "yesterday's living". The "torn-off senses" of the dead continue to sense and to be sensed, to feel and to be felt; in their very "absence" these "unknown dead" have an effect. In a way similar to the destroyed first moment of Stella and Robert's meeting – and, moreover, like Louie, who "felt she did not make sense, and still worse felt that the others knew it" – it is not, however, "their death" which "reproached those left living", but rather, "their unknownness" (*ibid.*, 165). In this novel (*ibid.*, 100), and in one of Bowen's essays of the Blitz, "London 1940", strangers bid one another "goodnight, good luck". Worse than simply "to die that night" is "to die unknown".[21]

Mourning, the means by which one accepts the loss of a love object, cannot occur here precisely because of this "unknownness". Unmourned, the dead continue to haunt the living, to "reproach" them with their unknowability, with the unincorporated psychic gap they figure. If it is the case that trauma is "about *not knowing* the extent of horror that one faces", and moreover, that trauma returns precisely because it was "unassimilated", because it was "*not known* in the first instance", then it might be seen that the unknown dead of *The Heat of the Day* call attention to the way in which trauma, the unknown, resists comprehension and evokes fear.[22] "I tremble", states Derrida, "at what exceeds my seeing and my knowing".[23] For Stella and Robert to mourn their unknown dead moment, then, may be one way of approaching a modern mourning of thousands of unknown dead people, those "Uncounted … shoals" which overwhelm their capacity for grief, their deaths part of "the even worse you could not be told and could not desire to hear" (*HD* 100).

But it is precisely in seeking to be known by another that Stella incorporates the horrific unknown into her own identity. Stella's traumatic discovery is concerned with more than, as Julia Briggs notes, "the theme of the impossibility of knowing another human being".[24] Her relationship with the traitor Robert, the conflation of her life with his, means that even as Stella insists on their "knowing" (*HD* 100) one another, Robert's unknownness has become, in Jordan's terms, "a shadowy side of herself",[25] "*without* [*her*] *knowing*" (*HD* 130; emphasis added): as Robert insists, "there's been you and me in everything I have done. – You can't see that?" (*ibid*, 304). In fact,

[21] Bowen, "London, 1940", 24.
[22] Caruth, *Unclaimed Experience*, 4 (original emphasis); Hepburn, *Intrigue: Espionage and Culture*, 147 (original emphasis).
[23] Derrida, *Gift of Death*, 54.
[24] Julia Briggs, "Resisting Nostalgia, Elizabeth Bowen's *A World of Love*", in *Women's Writing, 1945-60: After the Deluge*, ed. Jane Dowson, Houndmills: Palgrave Macmillan, 2003, 30.
[25] Heather Bryant Jordan, "A Bequest of Her Own: The Reinvention of Elizabeth Bowen", *New Hibernia Review*, XII/2 (Summer 2008), 50.

Robert's unknownness is so penetrating that Bowen's novel has been accused of inadequate characterization by several critics.[26]

The boundaries between self and other, ally and enemy, have collapsed; Stella and Robert are, "in effect … one another's accomplices already" (*HD* 192) because, Ellmann points out, Stella "has been practicing neutrality involuntarily. Knowingly, she has been working for the Allied cause", while "unknowingly, she has been sleeping with a Nazi spy".[27] Unnoticed, Stella has been psychologically infiltrated by – and has become (one of) – the unknown. That "wall between the living and the dead [has] thinned" and it is no longer so easy to tell the living self from those unknown dead (*HD* 99-100). Robert, the wounded returned soldier of the First World War, animates the spectres of the war dead and comes to figure a locus of trauma and of traumatic effect, "the delayed effects of strain or shock" (*ibid.*, 343). But more than this, Robert comes to signify the unknown, unseen, or unrecognized site of trauma within Stella's psychic structures. As "His experiences and hers became harder and harder to tell apart", and "everything gathered behind them into a common memory" (*ibid.*, 108), comes the traumatic recognition, for the reader and for Stella, not just that, as Hepburn states, "the beloved face belongs to a spy",[28] but that Robert's behaviour is no longer only a "malady" of his (*HD* 310). Stella's body has become the site of the traumatic element; the "infestation" (*ibid.*, 311), the infection of the traumatic past has been caught, unknown, by her.

Spectral effects

The narrative structures of the traumatic unknown in *The Heat of the Day* enact a relationship between the modern discourses of psychoanalysis and cinematography. Indeed, the novel's engagement with the unknown is conditioned by spectrality and performance in terms of its characterization and as a function of the Modernist narrative itself. *The Heat of the Day* works to underscore its sense of

---

[26] For example, Bernard Bergonzi, *Wartime and Aftermath: English Literature and Its Background, 1939-60*, Oxford: Oxford University Press, 1993, 87; Lis Christensen, *Elizabeth Bowen: The Later Fiction*, Copenhagen: Museum Tusculanum, 2001, 165; Corcoran, *The Enforced Return*, 188; Ellmann, *The Shadow Across the Page*, 160; Jordan, *How Will the Heart Endure*, 156.

[27] Ellmann, *The Shadow Across the Page*, 152.

[28] Hepburn, *Intrigue: Espionage and Culture*, 164.

the traumatic unknown and of façade through its self-conscious engagement with cinema, photography, and fiction, and with the ghostliness of these mediums. During the twentieth century, Luckhurst argues, the new stylistic devices which cinematic technology made available – in particular, conventions to mark temporal disruption, such as the flashback – made cinema "a cultural form closely attuned to representing the discordances of trauma"; so close, indeed, that it helped to "shape the psychological and general cultural discourse of trauma".[29] *The Heat of the Day* makes use of cinematographic metaphors as a means of elucidating the ways in which trauma is (re)produced in narrative. In "Notes on Writing a Novel", written during the war, Bowen makes a direct link between cinematic devices and the novel:

> The cinema, with its actual camera-work, is interesting study for the novelist. In a good film, the camera's movement, angle and distance have all worked towards one thing – the fullest possible realization of the director's idea, the completest possible surrounding of the subject. Any trick is justified if it adds a statement. With both film and novel, plot is the pre-imperative. The novelist's relation to the novel is that of the director's relation to the film. The cinema, cinema-going, has no doubt built up in novelists a great authoritarianism. This seems to me good. (*PC* 184)

In *The Heat of the Day*, cinematic metaphors are, overwhelmingly, associated with Robert: if he is seen, as I have argued, as the locus or the continuing effect of trauma in the novel, then the use of cinema's stylistic devices enable his traumatic representation. For example, in the lounge at Holme Dene, which appears to have "the glossy thinness of celluloid" (*HD* 124) Robert looks, in the late afternoon light, "like a young man in Technicolour" (*ibid.*, 125). Earlier, Stella wonders if he is "fictitious" (*ibid.*, 106). But it is the stilled image of him with "his thumb on his lighter", stilled in the same way that "in the cinema some break-down of projection leaves one shot frozen, absurdly, on to the screen", which figures, for Stella, "the face of before she opened her eyes" (*ibid.*, 106) to the "tingl[ing] … shock" of "the breaking down of immunity" (*ibid.*, 101). The freeze-frame thus comes to

[29] Luckhurst, *The Trauma Question*, 177.

figure the destruction of cinematic, romantic, and of defensive illusion. The traumatic recognition or "apprehension of loss" (*ibid.*, 105) describes, for Stella, the sudden end to her "immunity"; she moves from being the detached "onlooker" (*ibid.*, 102) to experiencing the effects of the traumatic event, a feverish "nervosity" figured as "a sort of imprisoned humming" in her head (*ibid.*, 101).

These aspects of the novel are also qualified by its Modernist concern with psychoanalysis – most clearly in terms of seeking Robert's "case-history" (*ibid.*, 112) and his motivation for betraying his country. In this way, *The Heat of the Day* may be seen to anticipate the Derridean equation concerning cinema, psychoanalysis, and spectrality. For Derrida, as for Bowen, the ghost and the actor are aligned. Playing himself in the film *Ghost Dance* (1983), and asked for his opinion on the existence of ghosts, Derrida responds:

> Curiously, instead of playing myself, without knowing it I let a ghost ventriloquize my words, or play my role .... The cinema is the art of ghosts, a battle of phantoms .... It's the art of allowing ghosts to come back .... All this, it seems to me, has to do with, with an exchange between the art of the cinema, in its most original, unedited form and an aspect of psychoanalysis. Cinema plus psychoanalysis equals the Science of Ghosts.[30]

In the context of *The Heat of the Day*, the notion of "playing oneself" is curious: although Harrison, the counterspy, is notably described as a "ghost or actor" in terms of his "appearances" (*HD* 155), he is not the only character who is figured in this way. Stella, for example, preferring to "sound a monster than look a fool", for years performs the role of the *femme fatale*, the guilty party in her divorce from Roderick's father, Victor (*ibid.*, 251). Indeed, she is first seen "mim[ing]" an "idiotic play at the window" (*ibid.*, 20) of her flat, framed like an actress by the blackout curtains which open on this "theatre of war" (*ibid.*, 348). Her flat is let already furnished, so that "surrounded by somebody else's irreproachable taste", she inhabits a space unmarked by her own preferences (*ibid.*, 22). And even at the inquest into Robert's death, she appears, in character, "as the woman friend in the luxury flat" (*ibid.*, 340). This means that in much the

[30] Jacques Derrida, in *Ghost Dance*, dir. Ken McMullen, Other Cinema (1983).

same way as Derrida describes, Stella does not play herself, but rather allows a "ghost" to "ventriloquize [her] words, or play [her] role". In so doing, the novel exposes "Stella" as signifying an identity as tenuous, as unknown, as that of "Harrison", who similarly "guy[s] himself" (*ibid.*, 12). Thus, when Stella longs to stay "forever" at Mount Morris, "playing this ghostly part", and "Unwillingly" regards "her gloves, shaped by her hands, her bag, containing every damning proof of her identity, [which] were still, always, there on the centre table where she had put them down", what she longs for is to play the ghost, rather than to allow the ghost to play her, to continue to shape and play out the set of expectations – what she "always" does – that make up "Stella" (*ibid.*, 182).

The Heat of the Day's associations between spectrality and identity make a subtle but powerful statement about the threat war and trauma pose to consistency of character and psychological stability. This novel posits another implication of the Derridean equation of cinema and psychoanalysis, precisely because of the way in which cinema – and, by extension, other performative media, such as fiction and photography – participates "in the process of haunting which, by itself, deconstructs life/death, presence/absence and being/ nonbeing".[31] The photographs which cover the walls of Robert's childhood bedroom "empty" the room of its occupant's existence, in the past and in the present:

> "Each time I come back again into [this room] I'm hit in the face by the feeling that I don't exist – that I not only am not but never have been." ….
>
> "But what were you doing *then* – and *then* – and *then*?" she asked, pointing from photograph to photograph. "Or at any rate, who was doing what you seem to have done?"
>
> "You may ask. I not only have no idea now but must have had even less idea at the time." ….
>
> "– Still, those must once have been moments."
>
> "Imitation ones. If to have gone through motions ever since one was born is, as I think now, criminal, here's my criminal record. Can you think of a better way of sending a person mad than nailing that pack of his own lies all round the room where he has to sleep?" ….

---

[31] Louis-Georges Schwartz, "Cinema and the ~~Meaning~~ of 'Life'", *Discourse*, XXVIII/2-3 (Spring/Fall 2008), 13.

> Comfortably slipping her arm through his, she said: "No, they've only made this room as though you were dead." (*HD* 129; original emphasis)

These photographs testify to Robert's "criminal" performance or "Imitation" of existence, to his sense that the self is unknown, even absent, because it is ventriloquized and, like "Stella", constructed of "motions" carried out by a ghost, a *doppelgänger*. But what is most disturbing about the photographs, I think, is that even as the room forms a kind of memorial, this sense of Robert's death becomes a simile, or a performance of memorialization: recalling Portia's bedroom in *The Death of the Heart* (*DH* 106), the room works "*as though*" Robert were dead, and thus comes to figure a doubled performance of his death, recording his non-existence or unknownness in the past, and enacting it in the present.

The room seems to indicate that Robert is neither living nor dead, so that he comes to exist only on the spectral border between the two. This kind of performance also describes Cousin Nettie's madness; unable to live up to Francis' expectations of her role as his wife, she "took to going nowhere but up and down stairs, till I met my own ghost" (*HD* 242). Nettie, like Robert, plays out her role until she is faced with the shuddering of her own identity, and recognizes that this role has been played by a ghost. If this kind of performance provokes in both Nettie and Robert a psychological collapse, then it might be seen that the novel anticipates a similar fate for Stella. Indeed, her final announcement to Harrison that she is to be married to "a cousin of a cousin" (*ibid.*, 363) suggests that she may be caught in a repetition of, haunted by, the fate of Cousin Nettie. To meet one's ghost is thus a traumatic confrontation with one's own future and, moreover, with one's own death. To meet one's own ghost is an uncannily Modernist confrontation with the simultaneously known and unknown self.

Falling effects

The hauntedness of these characters, this psychological embedding of their own deaths, thus figures a means of approaching the unknown: that is, trauma, which "can be grasped only in the very inaccessibility of its occurrence".[32] ("One doesn't know *why one trembles*.") This inaccessibility or unassimilability, Caruth states, is constituted, in Freud's explanation of trauma in terms of a train accident (in *Moses and Monotheism*), through "*the act of leaving*"; this trauma, "its very unconsciousness", she adds, "is borne by an act of departure". But more than this, Caruth asserts, Freud's example "is laced in the German" with variations upon the word, "*fallen*, 'to fall'": "Between the *Unfall*, the accident, and the 'striking' of the insight, its *auffallen*, is the force of a fall, a falling that is transmitted precisely in the unconscious act of leaving."[33] This analysis constitutes a useful means of understanding trauma in terms of the unknown and the effects of the unknown in Bowen's wartime novel as it elucidates the event of Robert's death, his "fall or leap" from Stella's roof. The act of falling, that figuration of death, destruction and decay which recurs throughout this novel (recall the falling leaves and the falling bombs), may be seen to parallel the psychological behaviour prompted by the traumatic event. That is, extending Caruth's analysis, it might be possible to consider that the initial fall (the *Unfall*) constitutes the accident, or the initial traumatic event; the falling itself constitutes the period of latency in which gathers "the force of a fall"; and the landing (the *auffallen*) constitutes a figuration of the impact or effect of the event. The first two stages can only be experienced through the anxious recollection of the third; it is for this reason, perhaps, that Robert's death is only narrated in terms of its impact and its aftermath. Stella "never, then, *was* to know what had happened" (*HD* 340; original emphasis).

Even in Stella's testimony, the temporal gap between Robert's departure from her flat and her discovery of his body cannot be narrated:

> No, I had not heard anything: I simply went down .... I went down and opened the street door .... I say, I simply went down. No, nothing made me: I simply thought I would go downstairs and look out of the door. I don't know why: why does one do anything? .... I beg your pardon .... No, I don't know how long after: I didn't look at the clock. Two minutes, five minutes, ten minutes: I don't know. (*Ibid.*, 341)

[32] Caruth, *Unclaimed Experience*, 18.
[33] *Ibid.*, 22 (original emphasis).

Between the fall and the impact – in echo of that "shaft of anticipating silence" through which falls the bomb that demolishes the first moment of Stella and Robert's meeting – thus lies the force of the fall, the force of the unknown (*ibid.*, 104). This is figured not only through Stella's inability to answer the questions posted at the inquest – "I don't know" – but through the ellipses which at once form a structural fragmentation of her testimony and mimic the psychological inaccessibility of the traumatic event. And the trembling impact of Robert's fall also reaches Louie; but because for her the identity of the faller is unknown, she imagines the faller as Stella:

> For Louie, subsidence came about through her now knowing Stella not to be virtuous .... For her, therefore, now it was Stella who had fallen into the street. (*Ibid.*, 344-45)

That "subsidence" in Louie refers to part of the opening sentence of the chapter, in terms which again place emphasis upon a quaking or trembling: "There can occur in lives a subsidence of the under soil" (*ibid.*, 339). It is, then, Louie who feels the impact, "the long-term effects", of Stella's fall, because it is precisely as a consequence of her sense of Stella's lack of virtue (as a "fallen woman") that Louie, "unknown" to Connie, "drop[s] back again into vagrant habits", and becomes pregnant with her child (*ibid.*, 346). The infant Thomas Victor upon whom the novel closes is thus himself a traumatic effect, the trembling force of the fall as it is felt.

Secret effects

The Heat of the Day engages with what I see as a recurring idea in Bowen's fiction: the relationship between literature, secrecy, and the memory of trauma. Specifically, it seems to me that in *The Heat of the Day*, secrecy is embedded as a traumatic event in the novel's idealization of narrative:

> [Stella] looked from the armchair proper to Robert to the armchair commandeered by Harrison, but found herself thinking of neither of these – of, rather, Victor, her vanished husband. Why of Victor now? One could only suppose that the apparently forgotten beginning of any story was unforgettable; perpetually one was subject to the sense of there having had to be a beginning *somewhere*. Like the lost first sheet

> of a letter or missing first pages of a book, the beginning kept on suggesting what must have been its nature. One never was out of reach of the power of what had been written first .... The beginning, in which was conceived the end, could not but continue to shape the middle part of the story, so that none of the realizations along that course were what had been expected, quite whole, quite final. (*Ibid.*, 146; original emphasis)

In Stella's reverie, the secret or unknown narrative beginning takes on the characteristics of the traumatic event – felt only in its impact, in its power to "shape" successive "part[s] of the story". The emphasis on an unknowable "*somewhere*", moreover, articulates the "*something*" which comes, in the novel, to figure the inaccessible secret of Robert's psychological trauma, which has the explosive potentiality of "dynamite" (*ibid.*, 67; see also 32, 143, 213, 303, 337, 358). The "something, somewhere" is the unknowable traumatic event, the unassimilable secret.

But above all, the passage draws attention to the strange paradoxical forgetting of the unforgettable, the way in which trauma is at once preserved and inaccessible, so that the story's beginning, which one did not have "time to know", remains unknown, even as its effects are felt (*ibid.*, 358). This is finally recognized by Stella as a coping mechanism when she observes to Harrison:

> Yet most of all there is something one has got to forget – that is, if it is to be possible to live. The more wars there are, I suppose, the more we shall learn how to be survivors. (*Ibid.*, 358)

Forgetting, the embracing of the unknown, is finally acknowledged as a condition of wartime, and of modern, survival; trembling, "an experience of secrecy or of mystery", is *The Heat of the Day*'s testament to this.[34]

[34] Derrida, *Gift of Death*, 54.

CHAPTER 7

POST: *A WORLD OF LOVE*

> "Reading a letter, only." Jane hesitated, put up a hand and glanced at it, as though wondering whether it should or should not have sealed her mouth. But she *was* glad to have spoken. "One of some letters," she said, beginning to smile.
>
> "What, then the post's come? What have they done with mine?"
>
> "Not the post. No, these came out of a trunk." (*WL* 26; original emphasis)

> Let us note: *Nachtrag* has a precise meaning in the realm of letters: appendix, codicil, postscript. The text we call present may be deciphered only at the bottom of the page, in a footnote or postscript. Before that recurrence, the present is only the call for a footnote.[1]

A World of Love is circumscribed by letters, but these letters are "not the post", not what they appear, or purport to be. They are purloined letters: returned to sender, put aside, put inside a trunk, and disinterred by another. The seal – of the trunk, of the letters, of Jane's mouth – is broken, and the letters are revealed to be "not the post" just delivered, but the past, unearthed from its archive. This narrative of purloined letters opens up ideas about the siting of memory, the ownership and theft of identity and of a text, and about the question of textual privacy. In this chapter, I will consider the ways in which the letters of *A World of Love* disrupt conventional notions of time and space by analysing the novel in terms of Kristeva's essay "Women's Time", and in terms of Derrida's motif of *destinerrance* as part of Bowen's exploration of the strange structure of trauma's emergence in the present.

---

[1] Jacques Derrida, "Freud and the Scene of Writing", trans. Jeffrey Mehlman, *Yale French Studies*, XLVIII (1972), 93.

In the shadow of the obelisk posted before the front door, and beneath the letters in the attic, the Danbys live as uncertain tenants of Montefort, Antonia's crumbling property and a symbol of the Anglo-Irish "descendancy". Fred Danby is Antonia's illegitimate cousin, charged with the care of the house, the farm, and Lilia, once fiancée of Fred and Antonia's cousin Guy, who himself was one of "a generation … mown down" in the First World War (*WL* 44). Abandoned to a life together, Fred's "unforeseen passion for [Lilia] ran its unspeaking course"; now the couple and their two daughters, Jane and Maud, live in a quiet, tense isolation behind locked gates (*ibid.*, 18). The events of the novel fill only two days, but they compact a stillness and endlessness that has haunted Montefort since Guy's death decades earlier; time stretches out the lengthy summer days in one pregnant pause: "the house was great with something" (*ibid.*, 27), caught, as it were, between the strokes of the kitchen's stopped clock (*ibid.*, 21). Antonia and Jane, both back from London, stir up memories in ways resented by Lilia, the "snow-woman" (*ibid.*, 18) frozen in time, her anaesthetized resolve melting beneath the oppression of the "heat of the day before" (*ibid.*, 9).[2] Lilia has "seceded from life"; she has become "marble", and "set up as a statue" (*WL* 96). She thus recalls Anna Quayne in *The Death of the Heart*, for her heart is atrophied, numbed in response to the trauma of failed romantic love. The novel's action concerns Jane's discovery (or theft) of a cache of love letters in a trunk in the attic – dateless, unaddressed letters thought to be from Guy, passed from hand to hand throughout the novel, and provoking in each woman the hallucination of Guy's presence (*ibid.*, 41).[3] The penultimate event of the novel, like the conclusion of Bowen's only other novel set entirely in Ireland, *The Last September*, is a conflagration: Jane burns the letters, Guy's post.

---

[2] For further discussion of "heat" in *A World of Love*, see Bennett and Royle, *Elizabeth Bowen and the Dissolution of the Novel*, 106; Christensen, *The Later Fiction*, 91; Ellmann, *The Shadow Across the Page*, 186; and Martha McGowan, "The Enclosed Garden in Elizabeth Bowen's *A World of Love*", *Eire-Ireland*, XVI (Spring 1981), 55.

[3] This spectral character is not typical of Bowen's novels, but is the "closest she came to writing a ghost novel" (Ellmann, *The Shadow Across the Page*, 182), and "to the explicit supernaturalism of some of her short stories" (Neil Corcoran, "A Ghost of Style: The Aftermath of Anglo-Ireland in Elizabeth Bowen's *A World of Love*", *English*, LII [Summer 2003], 127). See also Lee, *Elizabeth Bowen*, 184.

Not the past

While it might be seen that *A World of Love* describes a movement from the timelessness of the unconscious and the latency period associated with the memory of trauma to an acceptance of linear time that represents an ordered past, present and future, far from being time*less*, the novel presents an alternative temporality to describe the structures of traumatic memory.[4] The novel is characterized by delay, by its sense of being "afterwards": post-Guy, post-war, post-Ascendancy. However, one of the paradoxes of remembering trauma is that time after, time post-trauma, fails to progress in a linear manner, but is rather compelled or condemned to repeat the past. The pause of latency that characterizes the deferred action of traumatic memory makes "post" a lie. Just as the letters of *A World of Love* are "not the post", the novel's sense of "afterwards" is also an illusion, for Guy's spectral presence means that life at Montefort can never be "post". Old calendars and the "often stopping of the cheap scarlet clock" in the Montefort kitchen "spoke of the almost total irrelevance of Time, in the abstract" (*WL* 21). But if linear "Time" is of "almost total irrelevance" here, an idea which is reinforced by the "datelessness" of the letters being attributed to "the count of time … being kept in some other way", then these texts – the novel and its letters – are not timeless, but rather work on their own temporal terms (*ibid.*, 34).

That is, the narrative is only timeless if we adhere to a conventional notion of linear temporality; the novel foreshadows Derrida's observation on the "timelessness" of the unconscious as "determined only in opposition to a common concept of time, a traditional concept".[5] The unconscious, Derrida argues, is "timeless only from the standpoint of a certain vulgar conception of time".[6] *A World of Love* derides the experience of remembering as a "going back", for it appears to experiment with thinking about memory and

---

[4] Christensen, for example, makes much of the timelessness at Montefort (*The Later Fiction*, 112, 152, 157). See also Rachel Mayrer, "Gothic Memory and Forgetfulness in Elizabeth Bowen's *A World of Love* and 'The Demon Lover'", *Irish Studies Review*, XVI/1 (February 2008), 34, 37, 40; and Josette Leray, "Elizabeth Bowen's *A World of Love*", in *The Big House in Ireland: Reality and Representation*, ed. Jacqueline Genet, Kerry: Brandon, 1991, 171.

[5] Derrida, "Freud and the Scene of Writing", 96.

[6] *Ibid.*, 97.

the unconscious as sites outside of "a certain vulgar conception of time", resisting linear notions of past, present and future. If traumatic memory refuses to see the past as past, then *A World of Love* stages this refusal of linear temporality, and instead posits not timelessness, but an alternative temporality of the unconscious, and of the novel as its symbolic figuration.

In resisting the measures of linear time, *A World of Love* moves away from such constrictions and towards cyclical and monumental time, a temporality which Kristeva has identified with the experience of the hysteric, the one who "suffers from reminiscences".[7] We might usefully read this novel in terms of a rejection of linear temporality, one that approaches Kristeva's description of the repetitive, cyclical, "extrasubjective" time of the hysteric. *A World of Love* enacts what Kristeva describes as "the massive presence of monumental temporality", a measure of memorializing "which has so little to do with linear time (which passes) that the very word 'temporality' hardly fits".[8] This conceptualization of time resonates, in particular, with the inescapable presence of the monument outside Montefort.

A World of Love cheats a linear conception of time, and figures monumental temporality as a more appropriate description of the way in which its time operates, a description already figured by the ivy, symbol of eternity, covering the house, as well as by what it calls the "poetically immortal" landscape (*WL* 48). *A World of Love* is not concerned to demonstrate the danger of a repressed past, but rather of the limitations of linear temporality. An inability to pin down time within a linear framework is repeatedly mentioned: for example, Fred and Jane observe that "This morning isn't this afternoon" (*ibid.*, 40), and "Yesterday feels like years ago" (*ibid.*, 55), while an indignant guest at Lady Latterly's dinner party tells Jane:

> Now it's no use trying to pin me down! When I say "one time," I mean the time I mean, and that's good enough .... I'm my own calendar. (*Ibid.*, 64)

---

[7] Julia Kristeva, "Women's Time", trans. Alice Jardine and Harry Blake, *Signs*, VII/1 (Autumn 1981), 17.

[8] *Ibid.*, 16. This suspicion of linear temporality in *A World of Love* prefigures the cryptic spatio-temporal structures of Bowen's next novel, *The Little Girls*.

The novel's task is not to exorcize the past, but to open out alternative temporal modalities, to reject an understanding of time that is solely linear, that is therefore "obsessional"[9] or "monomania[cal]" (*WL* 50).

Jane most powerfully resents the inexorable past of *A World of Love*:

> … she had an instinctive aversion from the past; it seemed to her a sort of pompous imposture; as an idea it bored her; it might not be too much to say that she disapproved of it …. Most of all she mistrusted the past's activity and its queeringness …. Yes, so far as she was against anything, she was against the past; and she felt entitled to raid, despoil, rifle, balk or cheat it in any possible way. (*Ibid.*, 35)

Jane's often-cited "aversion from the past", her "disapprov[al]" and "mistrust" of it indicate that it is impossible to confine the past to the past. Jane resents that such temporal limitations mean she is "required" to live in the "bad odour" of "Her time": "Like someone bidden to enter an already overcrowded and overcharged room, she paused for as long as possible on the threshold" (*ibid.*, 34). Jane's pause "on the threshold" postpones "for as long as possible" her acceptance of those temporal limitations. The stilled pose of this "inheritor" who figures "the foreignness of this supplanting new time" thus mimics the obelisk, the novel's sign of monumental time (*ibid.*, 51). Moreover, that obelisk signifies a shared site of spatio-temporal reference for Jane and Guy: monumental time does not insist upon their separation (*ibid.*, 35, 142). It rises "somewhat surprisingly" at the novel's beginning, to stand paused in thought, in Guy's thought, in Jane's thought, and is a reminder to pause for thought, to remember (*ibid.*, 9). Just as Jane pauses on the symbolic threshold, and pauses on the threshold of the novel, standing by the obelisk with Guy's letters in the novel's opening scenes, the temporality of *A World of Love* comes to rest, (re)poses, on the monument.

The obelisk is a symbol of monumental time, of perpetuity. It is a constructed site of memory, or *lieu de mémoire*.[10] It saves a spatio-temporal site for the act of remembering as it reminds one, in its pose,

---

[9] *Ibid.*, 17.

[10] See Pierre Nora, "Between Memory and History: *Les Lieux De Mémoire*", *Representations*, XXVI (Spring 1989), 7-24.

to pause. The obelisk, then, perpetually postpones the possibility of forgetting and functions as a permanent trace of memory. The monument holds the place of memory, and resists the way in which "life works to dispossess the dead, to dislodge and oust them" (*WL* 44). But the obelisk of *A World of Love*, as Fred and Lilia's response to it makes clear, fails in this task:

> "I wish I could remember its origin – surely it must have had one, didn't it, Fred?"
>
> "Chap put it up in memory of himself," said he, with a glance at the thing, for the first time struck by it.
>
> "What, while he was still alive?" marvelled Lilia. "Rather peculiar, surely? What was his name?"
>
> "Couldn't tell you."
>
> "Oh, then he *is* forgotten!"
>
> During the pause, Antonia joined the group, was asked, looked bored and supplied the name. (*Ibid.*, 137; original emphasis)

While the memorial does incite a "pause" in its observers, it is not a pause of reverent remembrance, but of absent-minded forgetting. Antonia steps into the breach of this psychic absence, "supplie[s] the name" and thus compensates for Fred and Lilia. But Antonia's act of remembering is a supplement to a memorial that was itself intended to act as a belated or deferred supplement to memory. More than this, insofar as the act of building a monument in memory of oneself suggests a fear of being forgotten, of being out of mind, it also comes to signify a site upon which one's identity depends, and is thus an extension of, or supplement to the self.[11] The obelisk of *A World of Love* in this way stands in for, holds the place of, the legitimate children the Danbys' ancestor failed to produce, children who would have borne his name and so prevent that name from being forgotten.

To cease to think about time in linear terms means that, rather than representing a ghost to be exorcized, Guy becomes an inescapably present figure of monumental time, and as immovably present as the obelisk. Indeed, for Josette Leray, the obelisk of *A World of Love* works as a guy for Guy; it figures "a double … a replacement that

---

[11] Mayrer suggests that the obelisk represents "forgetfulness", while the "forgotten family member is characteristic of the forgetfulness that seems to invade not the house but its residents" ("Gothic Memory and Forgetting", 34, 35).

signifies both the presence and absence of the dead man .... [It is] the anchoring point of Guy".[12] Thus, Antonia witnesses Guy, not so much as a ghost, conventionally conceived, but as he was and still remains:

> All round Montefort there was going forward an entering back again into possession: the two, now one again, were again here ....
>
> Their tide had turned and was racing in again .... This was not the long-ago, it was *now* or nothing .... Ghosts could have no place in this active darkness – more, tonight was a night which had changed hands, going back again to its lordly owners: time again was into the clutch of herself and Guy. Stamped was the hour, as were their others. What was returned to her was the sense of "always" – the conviction of going on, on and on ....
>
> They conceived of no death, least of all death-in-life – an endless rushing, or rushing endlessness, was their domain, as it was their element. (*WL* 77-78; original emphasis)

Antonia does not experience remembering as a return to the past, to the "long-ago", or as the past's return to the present, but as "the sense of 'always'". All "time" is an "endless rushing" of a turning "tide", measured only by cycles, by repetitions of "again", and the "on, on and on", of the monumental moon, with no regard for the march of linearity. All "time" is now, all time is "always", all time is "here". Time outside "now" does not exist: it is "nothing". A similar temporal collapse also occurs when Lilia perceives Guy's presence: when "The breathless girl stop[s] to put down the woman's workbox", Lilia is at once both girl and woman, undivided by a linear understanding of the person she has been and is now (*ibid.*, 98). Death, for Guy, is an impossibility, for this would require the passing of time, and in this site of "endlessness" – notably not "timeless", but "endless" – beneath the awe of the obelisk and of monumental time, Guy is always already present, immortal.

The desire for monumentalization, then, figures the desire for immortality, or what Derrida has conceived of as "archival desire".[13]

---

[12] Leray, "Elizabeth Bowen's *A World of Love*", 171-72. Ellmann also observes that "it is the dead that keep the living in position in *A World of Love*, indeed the word 'guy' means a rope, chain, or rod used 'to secure or steady anything liable to shift its position or to be carried away'" (*The Shadow Across the Page*, 180).

[13] Jacques Derrida, *Archive Fever: A Freudian Impression*, trans. Eric Prenowitz, Chicago, IL: University of Chicago Press, 1995, 12.

But even though the archive and the monument are sites of memory, paradoxically, Derrida states, such sites "will never be either memory or anamnesis as spontaneous, alive and internal experience". Rather, the archive, like the monument, works precisely "at the place of originary and structural breakdown of the said memory".[14] In *A World of Love*, the desire to resist being forgotten exhibited by the ancestor who built the obelisk is matched by Guy, who has, in a fit of archival desire before being sent to his wartime death, stored his letters in the Montefort attic. Both the monument and the archive are intended to remain and to preclude forgetting and the progression of linear time. And insofar as the archive is not, Derrida insists, "a question of the past", but "a question of the future, the question of the future itself", Guy archives the textual figurations of himself in order to exist in a future to come.[15] In its focus on the endlessness of futurity, the archive keeps its contents safe from loss and forgetting. This desire for monumentalization also describes Guy's designation of Lilia as his "intended", so that she too is determined by an event in the never-arriving future, an archive (or a world) of love for Guy. Linear time does not pass in the archive, in Lilia: it and she are sites of monumental time. The archive represents "always".

The archive or monument cheats the threat of death, of being erased or forgotten, and in this way works against the progression of linear time. But at every moment, Derrida asserts, the archive is threatened by the death drive, the desire to pre-empt destruction: this desire is "*le mal d'archive*, 'archive fever'".[16] Archive fever runs high in Montefort, as the novel persistently threatens conflagration, from Lilia's initial confession to Antonia that "I lie sleepless, sometimes, picturing you in flames" (*WL* 12), and Fred's insistence that the family clear out the attics and burn the contents (*ibid.*, 40), to a concern for the "stuffed, stuffy attics" (*ibid.*, 27), filled with the "inflammable" (*ibid.*, 40) "wreckage left by the past" (*ibid.*, 27). The "malady" which, the narrator observes, is peculiar to "Obstinate rememberers of the dead", is archive fever – a simultaneous desire to destroy and to survive (*ibid.*, 44).

---

[14] *Ibid.*, 11.

[15] *Ibid.*, 33-34, 36. See also Bennett and Royle, *Elizabeth Bowen and the Dissolution of the Novel*, 105.

[16] Derrida, *Archive Fever*, 12.

Not the post

By precluding the possibility of arrival, the novel's letters, those unsent missives, also communicate outside a conceptualization of linear time, and relate to Kristeva's monumental time, as "always". And just as the letters of *A World of Love* exist outside of linear temporality, they also resist space and destination. The novel's letters might be considered within the context of Derrida's "Envois", of the "irreducible twists in any sending system", and in particular, that which is "most private within such a system" – a love letter, for example.[17] The letters of *A World of Love* enact the possibility of what Derrida terms *destinerrance*, or adestination, described by J. Hillis Miller as "a spatial figure for time".[18] The letters and the obelisk thus both figure *A World of Love*'s concern with spatio-temporality. Derrida's notion of *destinerrance* describes the tendency of a letter to "wander", to "err" from the destination it "always fail[s] to reach", calling into question Jacques Lacan's assertion that "a letter always arrives at its destination".[19]

Referring to Derrida's essay, "Telepathy", in which he "hypothesizes a letter" sent into the world without a known receiver, Miller says of such a letter:

> Its content and its goal do not precede it. Someone or other chances upon the letter and says, "It is intended for me. It has chosen me, and I choose to be chosen by it. I say, 'It's me (*c'est moi*).'" That might seem to imply that the letter has found its intended recipient. No, the recipient did not exist before receiving the letter. The letter creates the recipient, unpredictably, incalculably, by chance or even by error. The letter reaches that recipient by *destinerrance*.[20]

The letters of *A World of Love* create Jane as the recipient, that unidentifiable "*YOU*". She insists that the letters have found her, chosen her, to have "been no more than delayed on [their] way to her"

---

[17] Alan Bass, "Translator's Introduction: L Before K", in Jacques Derrida, *The Post Card: From Socrates to Freud and Beyond*, trans. Alan Bass, Chicago, IL: University of Chicago Press, 1987, xii.

[18] J. Hillis Miller, "Derrida's *Destinerrance*", *MLN*, CXXI/4 (September 2006), 893.

[19] *Ibid.*, 897; Jacques Lacan, "Seminar on 'The Purloined Letter'", trans. Jeffrey Mehlman, *Yale French Studies*, XLVIII (1972), 72.

[20] Miller, "Derrida's *Destinerrance*", 905.

– reached, it seems, by a kind of romantic version of the "chance" or "error" of *destinerrance* (*WL* 48).[21] However, this is complicated by the fact that Jane has disrupted an archive. That is, although Jane fancies that she is the delayed but intended recipient of these letters, her fatal misreading of the purpose of these texts – that is, to immortalize Guy – means that she, like a grave-robber, purloins the documents from their attic-crypt. All the locks and knots of Montefort – the "chain-knot" on the gate (*WL* 116), Guy's signature, the knot of Antonia's pearls, Jane's ribbon on the letters – do little to hold off this act of theft.[22] Her appropriation brutally forces her mother to repeat the experience of traumatic loss (Guy's infidelity and death) as the letters, symbol of Guy, are first stolen and then burned in an audacious assertion of ownership brought about by *destinerrance*.

Jane raids and rifles through the attic and through her mother's memory, much as she also appears to have "ravened nothing but fairness out of her mother"; she mimics Lilia and her model of romantic femininity by resiting and re-entombing the love letters – under her pillow, within a ribbon, under a tree, under a stone – taking her mother's "world of love" for her own. "She likes to feel that they are [to her]", Antonia wryly observes (*WL* 43). Jane seems not to be in love with Guy, but rather in love with being her mother (who loved Guy): in love with being the "Beloved" (*ibid.*, 96). To be "Falling in love with a love letter" is to mimic Lilia, to be in love, to be in a world of love (*ibid.*, 39).

But Lilia's world of love is a world of loss, of nothingness, of death. Lilia is nothing other than "Guy's girl" (*ibid.*, 104), for "virtually, nothing more than this had happened to [her and Antonia] since their two girlhoods" (*ibid.*, 51).

> Yes, but if not the Beloved, what was Lilia, Nothing. Nothing was left to be.

---

[21] That the love letters are unaddressed, Clare Hanson notes, means that they "can seduce *anyone*: the Oedipal/romance script far exceeds any of the individual characters (the name Guy underlines this – the letters are from any man (guy) to any woman)" ("Little Girls and Large Women: Representations of the Female Body in Elizabeth Bowen's Later Fiction", in *Body Matters: Feminism, Textuality, Corporeality*, eds Avril Horner and Angela Keane, Manchester: Manchester University Press, 2000, 189 [original emphasis]).

[22] Christensen observes that Montefort is a "fortress" (*The Later Fiction*, 86).

> And now these letters. To whom, why?
> Are you to be leaving me nothing, O Guy, then? (*Ibid.*, 96)

Lilia is not only left nothing, willed nothing by Guy, but left as nothing, embodying the vacant crypt, the "O Guy", of Guy's archive.[23] Indeed, that "O" of "O Guy", symbol of his absence, reappears in Maud's obsession with the "o'clock", Jane's identification of herself as Ophelia, and in the novel's acronym, A.W.O.L., which links Guy's undesired absence with his military death. Jane, "her mother's daughter" (*ibid.*, 54), is similarly "mindless", nullified (*ibid.*, 18). Yet the mimic Jane does not say nothing, like her mother, but rather, says "nothing". Responding to Maud's desire to know what Jane is "playing" or "pretending", the elder sister replies, twice, "nothing", and when Maud fails to hear (*ibid.*, 47):

> "Nothing – nothing – nothing." On that descending note Jane again became as she was before, letting the deep keen dream come combing through her, keeping her being running like tressy water-weed, like Ophelia's drowned hair. (*Ibid.*, 49)

Jane is, like Ophelia, like Lilia, in possession of nothing but "husks" (*ibid.*, 34) of letters that are themselves "nothing" for, Lilia insists, "There happened to *be* nothing for Jane this morning" (*ibid.*, 37; original emphasis). Described by, in imitation of, and expressing "nothing", Jane embodies the generation Guy has failed to populate. "She should have been his daughter!" spills from Antonia's lips (*ibid.*, 80), just as Jane's confession that she had found the letters had earlier escaped from her unsealed mouth (*ibid.*, 26):

> "Poor Jane's said practically nothing."
> Lilia said: "It's been more than enough."
> "I only do wish," said the girl, "that I had said absolutely nothing …. From now on I shall; I mean I shall not." (*Ibid.*, 41)

---

[23] "That enchanting love-on-a-leave, that idealization undoomed – as he probably knew – ever to fade so far failed to connect in Guy with outside reality that he had forgotten to make a Will" (*WL* 14).

Yet saying "practically nothing", is not the same as saying "absolutely nothing" or, indeed, the same as saying the word, "nothing". Jane's unsealed mouth, forming the "O" of "nothing", speaks Guy's absence, and counters Lilia's cryptic silence.

Lilia's identity has been shaped by her refusal to mourn Guy's death. Indeed, *A World of Love* suggests that archive fever and melancholia amount to something very similar.

> Her inner face, by now gaunt with solitude, looked out not without nobility through the big white mask padded with flesh. Sorrow was there in front of her like an apparition: she saw now, with belated dread, what life had proved to be, what it had made of her …. Loss had been utter: not till today had she wholly taken account. Guy was dead, and only today at dinner had she sorrowed for him. (*Ibid*., 50)

Like Anna in *The Death of the Heart*, Lilia "mask[s]" and protects her "inner face", the youth she is paused in, and has never progressed beyond: "she still stood under that station clock. The clock-hands stood still: she was seventeen" (*ibid*., 95). Lilia is anaesthetized to "sorrow" until Jane pillages her memory, appropriates its contents, and betrays archival purpose by destroying that which has been carefully retained. Although Lilia believes that she has "stay[ed] faithful to Guy's memory", she has rather stayed faithful to her own memory, the memory of herself as she was in Guy's eyes, and thus to "Guy's memory" of her, stilled in time beneath that eternally striking clock (still striking, its chimes still sounding, thanks to Maud's obsession with Big Ben) (*ibid*., 17). And like Dinah in Bowen's next novel *The Little Girls*, the discovery that she has been robbed is devastating for Lilia; just as the "tearing-out of the centre of the picture still left a quiver of edges torn", the theft leaves behind a "quiver" of pain (*ibid*., 98). Lilia's numbness is disrupted by her daughter, who seeks to succeed to her identity, to survive her even before Lilia's death. Each time Jane rummages, as it were, in her mother's mind, Lilia appears to have difficulty breathing, clutching her hand to her throat or lungs as the parasitic girl reaps the fragments of her mother's life, wearing her down with the "intensity of a brought-about recollection" (*ibid*., 95; see also 42, 50, 90, 139).

Jane seeks to succeed – to purloin – her mother's identity. But theft is eventually re-enacted upon the criminal when the letters are stolen from Jane's imitation crypt. Acting on the assumption that it was Lilia who stole from her, Jane burns the letters, cruelly destroying that which signifies, indeed creates, the identity of the recipient, the identity over which she and her mother tussle: the "Beloved". Not only does the novel describe the traumatic loss of a lover, then, but the mother-daughter rupture, as Jane struggles to develop her own identity. Like Derrida's hypothetical letter, Jane, who is "seldom *addressed*" by her mother, enters the world without an "intended recipient" (*ibid.*, 38; emphasis added). The novel ends when, at the airport, a space that both is and is not a destination, and "with the air of someone who cannot help knowing she must be recognized", Jane reaches her lover by *destinerrance*, and "They no sooner looked but they loved" (*ibid.*, 149).

In her reading of *A World of Love*, Ellmann considers these problems of ownership – seen, for example, in Lilia's perturbed question, "How can they be 'from' when they're not *to* her?" – in the context of Lacan's "Seminar on 'The Purloined Letter'" (*ibid.*, 41; original emphasis).[24] However, where Lacan asks to whom a letter belongs, I want instead to consider where a letter belongs, thereby approaching Derrida's assertion that "the letter has … its own proper itinerary and location".[25] In Edgar Allan Poe's "The Purloined Letter" (1845), the "proper place" of the letter, the place in which "its meaning is found", Derrida asserts, is the "nothing[ness]" of woman, the Queen.[26] The letters of *A World of Love* – that never quoted space of nothingness – were thus best left in Lilia, site of cyclical time, who "queen[s] it" over Montefort (*WL* 18), whom Jane has, throughout the novel, sought to knock from her throne, and whom she plays at beside the river, repeating, "Nothing – nothing – nothing" (*ibid.*, 47). The "proper place" of the letters was not out in the open, but rather, in Lilia, in the nothingness, the nothing happening, of Lilia's past; yet once Jane has disinterred the letters, and set in motion the traumatic *destinerrance* of these texts, they can never go back: "ignorance cannot be made good" (*ibid.*, 119). Overcome by archive fever, Jane burns the letters so that they cannot be lost again; their only available

[24] Ellmann, *The Shadow Across the Page*, 182-84.
[25] Lacan, "Seminar on 'The Purloined Letter'", 57; Derrida, *The Post Card*, 439.
[26] Derrida, *The Post Card*, 439.

resting-place, now, is the "cave" of the kitchen range, not entombed but now cremated (*ibid.*, 21).

The obelisk functions as a site of monumental time, a notion of "always" that precludes the passage of linear time and thereby, of forgetting. So too, the preserved letters represent an archive, disinterred by Jane who, seeking to usurp Lilia's romantic identity, claims the place of recipient, destroying the possibility of Guy's resting-place in her mother's memory. The letters of *A World of Love* disrupt both preservation and anaesthetization to the past. These disruptions to spatiality and temporality enact a figuration of the Freudian *Nachträglichkeit*, the deferred action or afterwardsness characteristic of traumatic memory, so that the world of love woven by the delays and deferrals of these letters is representative of the alternative space and time, rather than the timelessness, of the memory of trauma. Yet the novel's conclusion is troubling because while Jane may have grown beyond playing at being in love, and is now able to look to (and love) the future, she has left the older generation, hapless victims of identity theft, caught in that monumental site, stilled before the house and in the backward glance of the two daughters. If, in *A World of Love*, the past is ultimately left behind by Jane, then Lilia, Antonia and Fred are left with it, denied the possibility of a working-through that, after the cremation of the letters, has been perpetually deferred.

CHAPTER 8

CRYPT: *THE LITTLE GIRLS*

> Yesterday, you may remember, we made each other a promise. I now recall it, but you already sense all the trouble we will have in ordering all these presents: these past presents which consist of the present of a promise, whose opening toward the present to come is not that of an expectation or an anticipation but that of commitment.[1]

> If alive but in hiding, the two should know they have nothing to fear from Dicey, who continues to guard their secret.[2]

The Little Girls, Bowen's penultimate novel, is a narrative concerned with a clandestine past; the novel's formal, thematic, and structural crypts at once protect and display its secrets. Committed to their shared "past present", the three women of this novel, three "Weird Sister[s]", return to the coffer or crypt they secretly buried together as three little girls (*LG* 176). It is their avowal to one another that links the two distinct temporal periods of the novel, and that ties Dinah ("Dicey"), Sheila ("Sheikie") and Clare ("Mumbo") together, as their divergent presents are linked by their commitment to a commitment of the past. In this chapter I consider how an understanding of the crypt as it is thought through in *The Little Girls* and as it has been theorized in contemporary critical theory are mutually enlightening. Not only do psychoanalytic and deconstructive theories of the crypt unpack this novel, but so too, *The Little Girls* encourages an interrogation and development of these very theories. Through an engagement with the

---

[1] Jacques Derrida, *Mémoires for Paul de Man*, trans. Cecile Lindsay, Jonathan Culler, Eduardo Cadava and Peggy Kamuf, rev. edn, New York: Columbia University Press, 1989, 47.

[2] Elizabeth Bowen, *The Little Girls* (1963), New York: Anchor, 2004, 29. Hereafter cited parenthetically as *LG*.

concepts underpinning cryptomimetic readings which, Jodey Castricano states, "[draw] attention to a writing predicated upon encryption", this novel deals with several questions surrounding the interaction of literature, trauma and memory.[3] *The Little Girls* complicates and disrupts the "return of the repressed", responses to trauma, and the representation of these in literature. Specifically, this chapter considers the ways in which *The Little Girls* is concerned with the representation of repression and its relation to non-linear temporality and chronology in narrative, as well as how this relates to the promises of the novel's plot, the interaction between identity and narrative, and the ways in which the crypt "opens up" an understanding of a "surface-depth model" of secrecy and literature. This not only moves towards an evaluation of the "ideal literary object", to use Miller's term, but more than this, to a consideration of what these cryptic structures, and their connection in this novel to criminality and patriarchy, might mean for our understanding of *écriture feminine*.[4] It elucidates how *The Little Girls* uses the crypt in order to think about surface and depth in narrative, and what this novel has to say about the nature of reading in Bowen, as well as about literature, or the ideal literary object, more generally.[5]

In the first section of *The Little Girls*, Dinah Delacroix collects objects for her large cave, or time capsule. Through these actions she recalls when she had, as a little girl, collected with two other little girls items intended for posterity. She seeks out her old friends so that they might together disinter their buried coffer of secret objects. These girls, now successful women, are reluctant to be unearthed in a manner so embarrassingly public, for Dinah has advertised widely and cryptically in order to find them; their reawakened friendship is tense and awkward. In the novel's second section, Bowen returns to the girls' childhood, to the burial of the coffer, and to the days leading up to the First World War. The third section returns to the present and the "[unburying] of the coffer" (*LG* 76). It is, however, discovered to be

[3] Jodey Castricano, *Cryptomimesis: The Gothic and Jacques Derrida's Ghost Writing*, Montreal: McGill-Queen's University Press, 2001, 6.
[4] J. Hillis Miller, "Derrida's Topographies", *South Atlantic Review*, LIX/1 (January 1994), 16.
[5] Ellmann, *The Shadow Across the Page*, 199; Bennett and Royle, *Elizabeth Bowen and the Dissolution of the Novel*, 135.

empty – a revelation which precipitates in Dinah something that might be called a nervous breakdown. The closing moments of the novel serve to reunite the three women in a relationship that was impossible while the coffer and its contents remained buried in their shared memory.

The box and the significance of its contents and later emptiness circumscribe the novel and its engagement with secrets and cryptic structure, despite Bowen's statement to the contrary in her notes for a public reading of *The Little Girls*:

> The "box" theme – *which I do hope may not be taken as* too *symbolic* is *far* from being the whole of *The Little Girls*
> It is, in fact, little more than the *spine* of the plot
> This is a story about identity.
> It is about the *involuntary* element in behaviour: "Chance, not choice."[6]

Dinah, however, advises that "you need not worry if it is a symbol, as practically everything is, as we now know" (*LG* 193). Nevertheless, while the "'box' theme" may not be "the whole of *The Little Girls*", it does form the "hole" of it, the cryptic silence around which the novel is built. By describing this theme as "little more than the *spine* of the plot", Bowen plays down this theme as the overarching structure or framework which holds together the novel as a "whole", but nevertheless is forced to admit the "fact" that it is "more than the *spine*". Indeed, the "'box' theme" at once encrypts and is encrypted by the "story about identity". Each woman's identity is as much tied to the existence of the coffer as its form and presence is a result of their identities. In structure and in content, *The Little Girls* reiterates these encryptions.

---

[6] Elizabeth Bowen, notes for a public reading of *The Little Girls* (n.d.), HRHRC 7.4 (original emphasis and punctuation). This concern with the underlying meaning of a symbol is also present in the earlier novels *The Last September* and *The Death of the Heart*; in the former, Lois and Marda express their exasperation that, in novels, "Even things like – like elephants get so personal" (*LS* 142), while in the latter, Eddie states that he "hate[s] art – there's always something else there" (*DH* 136).

Seizure and sensation

In *The Little Girls*, Bowen's experimentation with form and with objective narration mimics the structure of the crypt and the secret.[7] *The Little Girls* describes the composition of inside and outside: "people *are* much the same, if one goes down deep", Dinah observes; "All the variety seems to be on the surface" (*LG* 4-5; original emphasis). The novel's cryptic "Unknown Language" is a demonstration of the simultaneous possibility and impossibility of reading anything "outside-text", to use Derrida's famous injunction. Lis Christensen's identification of key word clusters, which reveal this novel's preoccupation with death and the supernatural, can then be used as a "positive lever" for a reading of the novel, without "designat[ing] either the word or the thing as the master key that will unlock the 'truth'".[8] In both form and content, the crypts or "Arkword[s]" (*LG* 272) of *The Little Girls* work to elucidate cryptomimetic reading.

"Two things are terrible in childhood", Bowen once wrote: "helplessness (being in other people's power) and apprehension – the apprehension that something is being concealed from us because it is too bad to be told."[9] Both "helplessness" and "apprehension" are concerned with the future, with being propelled along a passage of time, unable to stop its perpetual progression, anxious about the knowledge this forward movement might bring. Yet, Bowen suggests that it is knowledge of the past – specifically, a secret or unspoken past – that is feared. Apprehension or anxiety, as it was in my discussion of *The House in Paris*, is a derivative of helplessness, for in the act of traumatic clairvoyance, the child is frightened of that which she cannot control. In these ways, helplessness and apprehension are put to work in *The Little Girls*, for it is in part through an attempt to regain control that Dicey determines the "box possibility" (*LG* 113). It is Dicey's apprehension surrounding the unspoken secrets, the "transgenerational phantoms", as Abraham might term them, of her

---

7 Spencer Curtis Brown, "Foreword", in Bowen, *Pictures and Conversations*, xxxviii.

8 Castricano, *Cryptomimesis*, 7. Christensen identifies word clusters "revolving on death and burial … as well as those to do with the supernatural" (*The Later Fiction* 93, 95). See also June Sturrock, "Mumbo-Jumbo: The Haunted World of *The Little Girls*", in Osborn, *New Critical Perspectives*, 83.

9 Elizabeth Bowen, "Preface to *Uncle Silas*, by Sheridan Le Fanu" (1947), in *The Mulberry Tree*, 111.

deceased father and widowed mother that motivates her passion for the crypt, in her childhood and in her later life.[10] The reader's "demand for knowledge", and the text's demand that the reader engage with its secrecy, drive the narrative.[11]

Perhaps more explicitly than any of Bowen's other fiction, *The Little Girls* is a novel about memory, about the patterns of its preservation or abandonment: "the mechanics of nostalgia".[12] It is concerned with the ways in which memory, as in *A World of Love*, constitutes a space outside time: in Dinah's cave of memory-exhibits "it was some other hour – peculiar, perhaps no hour at all" (*LG* 5). The characters often insist on renaming memory, describing it as a "sensation" (*ibid.*, 20) or a "seizure" (*ibid.*, 44), precisely because of this lack of linear temporality, at best a confusion between past and present. Lee suggests that in this novel memory has "fallen into disrepute".[13] Rather, it seems to me that this novel demonstrates a suspicion not of memory but, as in *A World of Love*, of time and its linearity, since "Mere memory" is superseded by "sensation":

> I've been having the most extraordinary sensation! Yes, and I still am, it's still going on! Because, to remember something, all in a flash, so completely that it's not "then" but "now," surely *is* a sensation, isn't it? I do know it's far, far more than a mere memory! One's right back again into it, right in the middle. It's happening round one. Not only that but it never has *not* been happening. It's – it's absorbing! (*Ibid.*, 20; original emphasis)

These observations about memory recall the epigraph to this chapter, and Derrida's suggestion that "these past presents … consist of the present of a promise". The promise Dinah recalls "all in a flash" is still valid, still present – indeed, it has been all along. It is not a memory, for "it never has *not* been happening". Remembering the promise paradoxically introduces the impossibility of it as a memory

---

[10] Nicolas Abraham, "Notes on the Phantom: A Complement to Freud's Metapsychology" (1975), in Abraham and Torok, *The Shell and the Kernel*, 171.

[11] See Elizabeth Bowen, *Afterthought: Pieces About Writing*, London: Longmans, 1962, 218; and Ellmann, *The Shadow Across the Page*, 191.

[12] Marian Kelly, "The Power of the Past: Structural Nostalgia in Elizabeth Bowen's *the House in Paris* and *The Little Girls*", *Style*, XXXVI/1 (Spring 2002), 1.

[13] Lee, *Elizabeth Bowen*, 184.

or as past, and it is Dinah's acknowledgement of its continuing presence that precipitates her search for Sheila and Clare.

The structure of the novel underscores the continuity of "past presents", for as I argued of *The House in Paris*, the middle section of the novel is not presented as a flashback, but as "a separate narrative present".[14] Marian Kelly sees this middle section as "disrupt[ing] the forward motion of the text, forming a kind of black hole within it", a hole of stilled time into which Dinah is drawn.[15] Significantly, Dinah is "in the middle" of this sensation, "absorb[ed]" or even encrypted by it. The return of the past, Dinah's "sensation", is in a sense a haunting rather than a memory, for "haunting, by its very structure, implies a deformation of linear temporality" like that which she describes.[16] In fact, Clare observes that Dinah "never had any memory". Calling the act of remembering, instead, "a seizure", she implies an unexpected psychic spasm has collapsed the distinction between past and present (*LG* 44). It is, then, Dinah's climactic recognition of this temporal disintegration which incites her breakdown: "And now … the game's collapsed. We saw there was nothing *there*. So, where am I now?" (*ibid*., 208; original emphasis). Finally, the sensation or seizure is summed up by the discovery of there being "nothing *there*" – merely an empty coffer. When Dinah asks "where am I now?" (*ibid*., 104) she shows how this collapse means that she, as a "[cheat] of Time" (*ibid*., 8) is, like Edward in *Friends and Relations*, now unable to position herself temporally. Dinah's real question is: "*when* am I now?" This kind of uncertainty about space and time, the narrator asserts, "causes … anxiety" (*ibid*., 51).

However, while the past as revenant works in this text, as throughout Bowen's fiction, by means of the processes of traumatic memory, this novel twists the traditional means by which trauma and repression are thought about and represented. In *The Little Girls*, traumatic return is not constituted by the return of the past, since for one thing the coffer is empty, and for another, the "cave idea's … been really only a repetition. – No, perhaps not so much exactly that

---

[14] Christensen, *The Later Fiction*, 159.

[15] Kelly, "The Power of the Past", 3.

[16] Peter Buse and Andrew Stott, "A Future for Haunting", in *Ghosts: Deconstruction, Psychoanalysis, History*, eds Peter Buse and Andrew Stott, Houndmills: Macmillan, 1999, 1.

as a going back, again, to something begun" (*ibid.*, 21). Because the cave is an imitation of the coffer from Dinah's childhood, a repetition of an act from long ago, it is Dinah who has returned to the past – the past has not, by contrast, returned to her. This uncertainty about the activity or passivity of traumatic return, of the sense in which Dinah is both haunted and haunting, points up Bowen's deconstruction of trauma-time in her novels, and the ways in which she seeks to write and represent trauma in narrative.

By the novel's end, however, Dinah admits to Clare that "Mistakes have histories, but no beginning – *like*, I suppose, history?" (*ibid.*, 299). Repetitions stretch back endlessly, it seems. Dinah has revised her belief that she has returned "to something begun", and recognized that it is impossible to identify a beginning to this history: "there's nothing like talking over old times is there? Those, one never gets to the end of, still less the bottom of" (*ibid.*, 246). The novel finds symbolic representation of this timelessness in the unfolding images in the window of the picture shop in the Old High Street:

> All this was to be wondered at through two layers of glass – the picture's shops window's [sic] and the glass in the gilt or ebony frames. But the greater wonder was that, outside the pictures, there the Old High Street actually *was*. You could verify simply by turning round: there, it indeed remained – a magnified picture. So seeing it, one saw it for the first time .... Moreover, a portion of the Old High Street (that exactly across the way from the picture shop) reflected itself not only in the shop window but in the glass of these numerous pictures of itself. The reflection itself looked like a large painting. The gables, etc., were there twice over. (*Ibid.*, 121-22; original emphasis)

Reflected, depicted, magnified, repeated, the street reappears over and over. *The Little Girls* removes the possibility of identifying a beginning to these reflections, because the Old High Street, the originator of these repetitions, is now merely "a magnified picture". The girls see it "for the first time", then "twice over": each reflection is a painting, each painting a reflection. This becomes a figuration of the way in which time works in *The Little Girls*: beginnings are made impossible, voided, and as Bennett and Royle argue, this shows "an indefinite deferral back to a past which is empty, like a coffer".[17] *The Little Girls* radically suggests that we are only subject to repetition, that an originary event (or "primal scene") cannot be located, and indeed, that in this way repression and the means by which traumatic memory functions call into question linear temporality and narrative chronology.

Shadow, surface and secrecy

The Little Girls therefore subverts a more conventional "return of the repressed" narrative. Although Dinah's cave of memory-objects could be read as her compulsion to repeat the repressed memory of burying the coffer in her childhood, and Sheila and Clare are at first resentful of the repressed Dinah's return to their lives, along with her "Insinuations – malicious, insidious, mischievous, damaging", the most important event of the novel, the apocalyptic unearthing of the empty coffer, demonstrates that sometimes the repressed primal scene cannot be definitively identified or located (*LG* 45). The discovery of the empty coffer, symbol of the lost memory, therefore provokes in Dinah a psychological collapse which points to her not as a hysteric but as a "cryptophore".[18]

The hysteric, Abraham and Torok suggest, practises constitutive or dynamic repression – here, "the desire, born of prohibition, seeks a way out through detours and finds it through symbolic fulfilment".[19] The cryptophore, on the other hand, is characterized by the presence of what is commonly and metaphorically referred to as the tomb and the lock, an analogy also used in *The Little Girls*, for in answer to Dinah's query regarding the location of the girls' "Unknown Language", Clare replies that it has "Gone" into an "attic" in her head – "And the key's lost" (*LG* 199). Similarly, Sheikie – whose nickname encloses a "key" that her Christian name does not – is described as being "More barnacled over. Far, far more barnacled over than you or I are" (*ibid.*, 186). Such architectural envisioning of memory usefully informs a psychoanalytic reading of the novel. The tomb and the lock are more accurately termed preservative repression; here,

[17] Bennett and Royle, *Elizabeth Bowen and the Dissolution of the Novel*, 130.
[18] Abraham and Torok, "The Topography of Reality", 158.
[19] *Ibid.*, 159.

> … an already fulfilled desire lies buried – equally incapable of rising or of disintegrating. Nothing can undo the consummation of the desire or efface its memory. This past is present in the subject as a *block of reality*; it is referred to as such in denials and disavowals.[20]

The hysteric, therefore, manifests a secret desire on the surface, while the cryptophore keeps the "secrets of the tomb" locked in hidden depths (*LG* 300).

The Little Girls makes this a debate about the cryptonymy of the literary object, and its argument returns to the problem of the crypt itself: that is, is the crypt the structure or the hollow interior? Is literature, "the ideal literary object", formed by the words manifest on the page, or by its latent content?

> But what does the cryptic structure have to do with literature? It would seem that the ideal literary object would harbour no secrets. It would always be wholly accessible by way of the words.[21]

> The content of the novel is what affects us; and the content, because it expands in the reader's mind, may by far exceed what is stated in the actual writing – this, in fact, is one evidence of creative power.[22]

For Bowen, it is the "shadow" which makes a novel:

> There is much that the reader relies upon being told, therefore much of writing is bound to be informative – as to what is happening to whom, and where, and when. So much is the bone-structure of story-telling. Novel-writing, however, is more than that: it is when we come to the narrative's "why's" and "how's," the complex causes of action, the ripples of its effect, the shadowy ambience of the personality, that we touch what makes the essential *novel*.[23]

---

[20] *Idem* (original emphasis).
[21] Miller, "Derrida's Topographies", 16.
[22] Elizabeth Bowen, *Afterthought: Pieces About Writing*, London: Longmans, 1962, 216 (original emphasis).
[23] *Ibid.*, 217 (original emphasis). "Shadow" reappears in Bowen's description of the fleshing out of character: "Complete and detached as beings, they reveal, as beings do, complexities, inconsistencies, contradictions; and, through being three-dimensional, they take on shadow" (*ibid.*, 218-19).

Although Miller (via Derrida) convincingly makes the argument that a text cannot be more than itself – "*Il n'y a pas des hors-texte*" – Bowen appears to anticipate (and to question) these very ideas and, just as assuredly, to demonstrate that the story may exist beyond the words on the page as part of the infinite process of the deferral of meaning back to an empty coffer.[24] A novel *can* harbour secrets, Bowen suggests. Just as the crypt cannot exist without both its firm shell and its inner space, so too, the novel is formed by both the physical words on the page and their embedded endless significations.

In a contemporary review of *The Little Girls*, Anthony Burgess picks up on this importance of surface and depth in this novel, stating: "you will find that women have a better natural fictional equipment than men. They notice surfaces, which is what novels are made out of; they have a phenomenal semantic range when it comes to dealing with texture, colour and nuance of speech; being the primal order of creation, they *enclose* men and see through them."[25] Burgess' observations are intriguing in terms of a reading of crypts and of literary objects in *The Little Girls*, for he explicitly states that "surfaces [are] what novels are made out of", suggesting, by extension, that secrecy and textuality are mutually exclusive. At the same time, he appears to be invoking the epithet of woman-as-crypt, "the primal order of creation". There is a slippage here in the assumption that the crypt (novel, woman) is the surface, that which "*enclose*[*s*]", not that which is enclosed. There is also a suggestion here of enclosing or encrypting as a means of control; men, secrets, "shadowy ambience" are "repressed" in order to be fully known, in order for the façade, the surface, the secret, to be "see[n] through". However, *The Little Girls* disrupts such ideas about surfaces and secrets, always already anticipating a reading that might reduce an understanding of the literary object to either surface or depth, rather than a play between the two. Although, as Bennett and Royle assert, "novels are entrances designed to entrance, like the entrance to Clare's novelty gift shop", they also pull us in, make us want to investigate

---

[24] Jacques Derrida, *Of Grammatology*, trans. Gayatri Chakravorty Spivak, Baltimore, MD: Johns Hopkins University Press, 1976, 158.

[25] Anthony Burgess, "Treasures and Fetters", *Spectator*, 21 February 1964, 254 (original emphasis).

those novel(tie)s, the secret depths and wares.[26] This is, perhaps, to what Lee refers when she notes that Bowen's "last two novels are looking for a new kind of fictional language and method". In doing so, they "stir up qualms about the novel form itself", for this novel, and the novel form more generally, is stirred by these complications of surface and depth.[27]

Although the act of critical, historicist reading may be seen to parallel the act of opening the coffer or crypt and releasing what it contains so that the discovery of the text's secrets give satisfaction to the reader, if the text (the crypt) is found to be empty, as it is for the little girls, this invites the sublime *jouisssance* of reading and interpretation. "And now, nothing", Clare silently observes to Dinah. "There being nothing was what you were frightened of all the time, eh? Yes. Yes, it was terrible looking down into that empty box" (*LG* 306-307). The very emptiness of the box provides a symbolic and textual representation of the terror of confronting the traumatic past.

Shame and silence

One of the novel's secrets is a promise made by three little girls: a promise to each other, committing to a present silence, and a promise to the future, consisting of both a warning and a testimony to their existence. However, the girls' strict adherence to the terms of the promise – that it should be kept secret – makes it shameful. The guilt they feel for having transgressed the proprieties of being "good little girls" evolves into a self-sentencing of criminal guilt, so that the secret itself is remembered as a crime. Abraham and Torok term the secret, or the location of its burial, "Reality", and note that it "is born of the necessity of remaining concealed, unspoken. This means that, at the moment of its birth, Reality is comparable to an offence, a crime."[28] In these ways, criminality, fear of the law, of being outside the law of the word, taints the text.

The clandestine or criminal nature of the secret first appears in Dinah's advertisements seeking her friends, whom she wishes to

[26] Bennett and Royle, *Elizabeth Bowen and the Dissolution of the Novel*, 132.
[27] Lee, *Elizabeth Bowen*, 183.
[28] Abraham and Torok, "The Topography of Reality", 158.

disinter.[29] Believing the documents to be a Will, a legal document, Dinah's housekeeper, Francis, reads:

> Imperative Dicey confer with Mumbo and Sheikie. The past not so buried as it appears ….
>
> Whether married or otherwise or living under real or assumed names …. Crisis arisen ….
>
> Your former confederate Dicey seeks you earnestly, in connection with matter known so far only to us. Whole affair now looks like coming to light ….
>
> Where are Sheila Beaker and Clare Burkin-Jones, last heard of in Southstone? Anyone who can throw light on their disappearance is requested to contact their anxious friend, the former Diana Piggott. If alive but in hiding, the two should know they have nothing to fear from Dicey, who continues to guard their secret. Should they care to write, she will not reveal their whereabouts. Whatever the past, she would gladly see them. Write Box xxxx. (*LG* 28-29)

Dinah's cryptic language, her encoded message to her childhood "confederate[s]" circles the idea of a criminal or shameful act (note that in these advertisements she nowhere refers to herself as Dinah Delacroix, her current, respectable name). More importantly than this, however, in demanding to be read "between the lines", her advertisements reveal the very presence of the secret – stripping the secret of its secrecy, she all but gives it away. It is for this reason that Clare and, especially, Sheila, are so concerned by Dinah's advertisements; indeed, Sheila suggests that they position themselves on the side of the law and take legal action against this "widely spread innuendo" and veiled accusation of criminal activity (*ibid.*, 47). The girls are, however, caught by another cryptic aporia, for it would be a moral crime to break the promise, and yet the promise and its keeping are also, they believe, criminal.

Intriguingly, the repetition of "Write Box xxxx" at the end of each advertisement foreshadows the unnameable crypt, the box, later revealed. To write to "Box xxxx" is to write not to Dinah, but to the secret she guards. Thus, also present in Dinah's search for her friends and in Sheila and Clare's conversation is a concern for names ("real or assumed"), and especially, for protecting a good name, as Sheila seeks

[29] Bennett and Royle, *Elizabeth Bowen and the Dissolution of the Novel*, 121.

to do through the law, in the name of the law. Her name, maiden and married, is that to which she attaches most importance; emblazoned on boards "all over Southstone and through the area", her name denotes her social standing and her location (*ibid.*, 44). Clare, too, attaches success to the name of her *alter ego*, "MOPSIE PYE", and is anxious to protect her business from scandal (*ibid.*, 46). The pseudonyms, or nicknames, of their childhood serve to cast further secrecy and illegitimacy across the advertisements, but they later work to improve the girls' friendship by becoming a means of tying the present to the past. The girls' names also complicate our thinking about secrecy in this novel, for their *alter egos* – their childhood nicknames and their changed names in adulthood – have enabled them to disappear while still remaining present. That is, the names of the little girls allow them to be visible and invisible at the same time, to hide themselves in plain view, as it were, emblazoned across signs and billboards.

In this way, the novel moves towards a Derridean or surface conceptualization of the literary secret. "Literature keeps a secret which does not exist, in some way", Derrida argues:

> Behind a novel, or a poem, behind what is in effect the richness of a sense to be interpreted, there is no secret meaning to be interpreted. A character's secret, for example, does not exist; it has no thickness outside the literary phenomenon. Everything is secret in literature and there is no secret hidden *behind* it – there you have the secret of this strange institution *on the subject* of which, and *within* which I never stop wrestling .... The institution of literature recognizes, in principle or essentially, the right to say everything or to say without saying, and thus the right to the secret displayed as such.[30]

The simultaneous secrecy and visibility which surrounds naming in *The Little Girls* suggests that everything, in this novel, is at once secret and not secret, there and not there, safely buried and yet gone. It is this paradox which incites Dinah's psychological collapse upon finding the coffer empty, for it is the empty box itself which figures literature's "right" to say everything and nothing, to at once insist upon the presence of a secret coffer and then to show this to be empty.

---

[30] Derrida, *Paper Machine*, 162-63 (original emphasis).

Secrets, crypts, in *The Little Girls*, have a false bottom: they are transgressive and criminal.

This is not the only crime of the novel; for example, Dinah and Clare break into Frank's house, but to leave an item (a mask) rather than to steal anything. (The discovery is made here that Frank, too, hoards boxes, "lawyer's boxes", the contents of which are unknown [*LG* 239].) It is for fear of incrimination that Dinah refuses to leave a thumbprint on the wax with which the girls seal the coffer; like a careful criminal, she will not leave evidence behind. Disobeying Clare's command that "We can't burgle", Dinah steals her mother's pistol from a drawer (*ibid.*, 115). The girls trespass in the dead of night to bury the coffer and to unearth it years later, searching for a space to keep a memory that has, as Abraham and Torok put it, no "*legal burial place*".[31] Finally, they discover that in the manner of a grave robber, someone has trespassed upon their burial site and stolen the contents of their crypt. There is, in addition, a crime lurking behind the scenes, only touched upon in the text; it forms part of the novel's "shadowy ambience". This crime is the suicide and accompanying unnameable shame of Dinah's father who, scorning the gun in his household's possession, threw himself under a train. Juxtaposed with this crime is the moral crime of infidelity: the secret love affair between Mrs Piggott and Major Burkin-Jones.

These crimes are outside the scope of the text, but they nevertheless exist, and are to what Bowen refers when she writes that: "In short, the 'musts' and 'must nots' of effectual novel-writing entail embarkation, by the author, upon something far wider, deeper and longer than what, in print, *in statement*, he will eventually present."[32] Bowen suggests that the novelistic "*statement*", the legal testimony, cannot ever cover everything – it will always exclude "something", which will then appear as a textual "nothing", a cryptic silence. Just as a secret demands the exclusion of others from the knowledge of its existence in order for it to be a secret, so too, the secret itself is excluded from the text. The secret's content, as it were, is less important than the fact that the secret itself exists, and what the secret

[31] Nicolas Abraham and Maria Torok, "'The Lost Object – Me': Notes on Endocryptic Identification" (1975), in Abraham and Torok, *The Shell and the Kernel*, 141 (original emphasis).
[32] Bowen, *Afterthought*, 219 (original emphasis).

does, a point *The Little Girls* demonstrates in the way it reinscribes the secret of the little girls. As Abraham and Torok point out:

> All secrets are shared at the start. Hence the "crime" under consideration cannot be a solitary one, since it was turned into a secret. The "crime" points to an accomplice, the locus of undue enjoyment, as well as to others who are excluded and, by dint of this same enjoyment, eliminated. In the absence of a concept of infringement, the "crime" would entail no secret.[33]

The link between the secret and the crime demands the presence of those who are included – the accomplices – and those who are excluded, or kept in the dark. The secret, then, is not only encrypted, it is itself a crypt, a site for inclusion and exclusion.

The return of the secret, making present a promise of the past, functions as a legacy. The three women – who now personify the posterity envisaged by the three little girls – become the inheritors of the crypt, those to whom their precious "treasures" and "fetters" are willed (*LG* 147). The little girls deposit in their coffer, their vault, their savings or promises for the future. Their later discovery that these material objects have been withdrawn, however, leaves open a site for haunting, for the "ghostly inheritance" of the spectre of their childhood.[34] The impossibility of inheriting from oneself therefore incites the temporal collapse of traumatic experience.

Shelley, a shotgun and the sixth toe

All three girls inherit, are haunted by, not only the legacy of their childhood, but the lives of their parents. Clare applies her father's military organization to the management of her business, while Sheila inherits in a more tangible sense her father's wealth (signified, in part, by the matching partner to the buried coffer, which stands in her large house) and his business. She secures this ownership through her marriage to the son of her father's business partner, whom she inherits after the death of her first fiancé, her husband's elder brother. Dinah is bequeathed much of her mother's property but she is also heir, in a

---

[33] Abraham and Torok, "The Topography of Reality", 158.

[34] Castricano, *Cryptomimesis*, 9.

sense, to her mother's beauty, to which she is said to accede after the elder woman's death.

As a cryptophore, Dinah is a victim of what Abraham terms a "transgenerational phantom", an unspeakable ancestral secret of which she is unaware: "what haunts are not the dead", Abraham notes, "but the gaps left within us by the secrets of others".[35] Mrs Piggott leaves in Dinah a crypt which encloses her unspoken secrets and triggers their compulsive repetition: "Widows … run in families", Dinah observes (*LG* 249). More significant than Dinah's repetition of her mother's young widowhood, however, is the unspoken love affair which she shares with Frank, Major Wilkins. This relationship may be seen to unconsciously re-enact the clandestine passion of her mother and Clare's father, Major Burkin-Jones. Dinah's curious question to Clare, "Does it ever seem to you that the non-sins of our fathers – and mothers – have been visited upon us?" also appears to point up an awareness of the ways in which these inherited secrets – whether they were acted upon or not –have shaped and ghosted the lives of the three girls (*ibid.*, 240). "Although what haunts us is what we inherit", Castricano proposes, "the legacy is always contradictory. Derrida suggests that it takes the form of a double bind: secrecy and choice."[36] The secrecy inherent in this observation is made clear through the notion of transgenerational haunting; if one considers choice as its inverse, however, the power of the past for these women becomes even more significant, for they choose to return for their inheritance, they choose to value the legacy of memory. They have chosen to adhere to their promise, and thus the secret transaction remains valid. Yet, as I earlier pointed out, Bowen asserts that this novel is "about the *involuntary* element in behaviour: 'Chance, not choice.'" Is it by chance that Dinah recalls the secret promise of the girls' childhood? Choice and chance – an "involuntary element" – are not mutually exclusive. Rather, it is the influence of memory – the behaviour of preservative repression and a memory thought to be forgotten – which, while masquerading as chance, actually shapes, makes choices for, the text.

The sway of repressed memory and a secret past upon Dinah is not unlike that which affects her mother, Mrs Piggott. Indeed, it is in part

---

[35] Nicolas Abraham, "Notes on the Phantom", 171.
[36] Castricano, *Cryptomimesis*, 17.

Dinah's memories of her mother – or, more precisely, the traumatic memory of her death – which incites her passion for burial and disinterment. Both Dicey and her mother are haunted by memory; they have "spun round themselves tangible webs, through whose transparency, layers deep, one glimpsed some fixed, perhaps haunted, other dimension" (*LG* 93).[37] While this might be seen as a reference to the secrets of their life before arriving at Feverel Cottage, the suggestion that both are "haunted" by an "other dimension" provides further evidence of the transgenerational phantom. As Ellmann has so insightfully noted, both the content and structure of the novel form a crypt around the dead mother, so that the repeated entombments of *The Little Girls* "re-stage the process of psychic incubism or encryptment in which the lost object is entombed alive within the ego".[38] The absent presence of the First World War, part of the gap between the two time periods of the novel, forms a crypt that houses the lost, beloved mother and, to recall my discussion in Chapter 1, a kind of wounding of the text.[39] That is, although Mrs Piggott – who does "nothing by halves" – plays a relatively minor part in the text of the novel, she cannot be overlooked (*LG* 95). The value Bowen places on latent content and "shadowy ambience" is pointed up by the assertion that "To disturb Mrs Piggott once she was *in* a novel was known to be more or less impossible" (*ibid.*, 94). Mrs Piggott, the dead mother, is a dead weight in the crypt of *The Little Girls*:

> "Did you ever wish she was not there?"
> "Well –"
> "Did you ever hate her?"
> "My mother? No, never," Clare said. That was that.
> "*I* liked her," said Dinah. "She was nice to me, and friendly to Mother."
> Clare said vaguely: "Went out of her way to be." (*Ibid.*, 240; original emphasis)

---

[37] Mrs Piggott and Dicey plan that they will together "start on making a shell box" so that the construction of crypts and boxes is pointed to as a shared interest (*LG* 164).

[38] Ellmann, *The Shadow Across the Page*, 199.

[39] Ellmann sees the dead mother to be, as in *The House in Paris*, "incubed in the central flashback" (*ibid.*, 177).

Dinah's questions to Clare imply that she herself hates her mother, wishes "she was not there". It is precisely because of her love for her mother that she has encrypted her, and is unable to be rid of her. Also implicit here is the girls' knowledge of the secret affair between Clare's father and Dinah's mother, for Clare's final comment suggests that her mother, too, knew of her husband's infidelity, yet performed ignorance when confronted with his mistress.

Parents, in *The Little Girls*, function as both a connection to, and as the legacy of, the past. "*We are dead, and all our fathers and mothers*" (*ibid.*, 147; original emphasis); as they bury the coffer, the chant of the little girls at once mimics a funeral and a disinterment. The inclusion of their "fathers and mothers" in this vow, and the grammatical ambiguity which suggests that the fathers and mothers are not only dead like the little girls, but are themselves the little girls, is striking. In particular, Dinah's revelation of the secret object she placed in the coffer is tied to the "shadowy ambience" of her father and his early death. It is not until very late in the novel that Dinah confesses her unnameable object to be a gun she "robbed" from her mother's glove drawer (*ibid.*, 248). In terms of Oedipal structures, the implications of taking the gun, a phallic object she supposes to have once belonged to her father from its highly feminine hiding-place are clear enough; what I find more intriguing is why Dinah should choose this object for burial in the coffer.[40] In her burial of the gun, phallic substitute for her father's presence – "a thing no widow should be without" – Dinah may be seen to demonstrate her resistance to war and to a patriarchal order that threatens to destroy the idyll she shares with her beloved mother (*LG* 248). In burying or pushing aside the perils of war and of the father, Dinah also resists the inclusion of the man who represents both of these – the soldier, Major Burkin-Jones – within the mother-daughter family unit. Her rejection of the father and patriarchal law which decrees that the "'product' of sexual union, the child, shall belong exclusively to the father, be marked with his name", is later reiterated by her refusal of her name, changing "Diana" to "Dinah" once an adult.[41] Her childhood nickname, "Dicey", also betrays an underlying uncertainty not only about her own name, but the name of the father, for as Sheila wonders, "Supposing … she

[40] See also Hanson, "Little Girls and Large Women", 193.

[41] *Ibid.*, 171.

never did have a father, at the best of times?" (*LG* 41) and Dinah's only reply to the question "What's your father?" is a blunt, "He's dead" (*ibid.*, 111). The burial of the pistol is thus an attempt to erase this uncertainty from her background and in this way to subvert the idea of woman-as-crypt and to control the encroaching patriarchal order.

This resistance to the law of the father is also made evident by the "Unknown Language" in which the girls write their message to the imagined inheritors of the coffer. The cryptic letter to posterity is another instance of the ideal literary object and an example of *écriture feminine*, writing the bodies of the little girls into the future. Through the creation of their own language and a message written in Clare's blood – the ink of her female body – the girls seal the box with a feminine authority designed to contain the patriarchal symbols they place inside. The secret objects of the coffer signify their rejection and burial of this order. Dinah's pistol removes her father's symbolic presence from her relationship with her mother; Sheila's burial of a sixth toe removed at birth demonstrates her defiance of approved notions of feminine beauty; and Clare's copy of Shelley places out of sight a phallogocentric language which might influence her own practice of *écriture feminine*:

> Clare locked herself up again, more violently, into the Unknown Language, in a wedge-shaped box-room inside one of the gables, under a spike. The place was lit by panes of glass in the roof: when nothing but night came through those, she had to stop. Downstairs, she could have found a bit of candle. But downstairs was all party voices and, worse, laughter. (*Ibid.*, 145)

Clare encrypts herself "into the Unknown Language" and, like Laura in *The Last September*, in an aptly termed "box-room", imitating the later entombment of the letter itself.[42] She works under a phallic spike, signifier of a language exemplified by Shelley, as a reminder of that

[42] Francis, "unable to be in the Secret Service", also encrypts his secret writing twice over, writing it "in an unbreakable code" and then burying it "among the bowels of plumbing under the pantry sink" (*LG* 26). Mrs Piggott, too, buries a secret letter (the contents of which are never revealed) beneath her own body: "Mrs Piggott got off the sofa; chiefly to disinter a letter on which she'd till now sat. She put the letter away in her little desk" (*ibid.*, 102).

which she must escape. Clare refuses, however, to work by the light of a candle, or to explain her activity to her father, who "wouldn't" – indeed, couldn't – "understand" (*ibid.*, 145). Sheila and Dinah's fear that they too will not understand the message to which their names are signed means another promise is tied to this secret language: that is, Clare's vow that her words are as good as her word: "Don't invent it so's it's unknown to *us*, though: you swear and promise? We must know what what we have said is" (*ibid.*, 115; original emphasis). The three girls must trust one another's sincerity in a cryptic and exclusively feminine language.

Dinah, however, struggles with an insufficient language haunted by secrets, amendments and lacunae:

> For here (and certainly fresh since yesterday) was a wad of thin, crumpled sheets in her handwriting – scarred with erasures, corrections, inserts, loops, brackets, arrows, marginal scrabblings. And all (that was, to judge by the first glance) saying, or attempting to say, the same thing, here or there with omissions or variations. (*Ibid.*, 27)

While for Clare, words and tangible text are of the greatest importance in examples of Dinah's writing – the drafts of her newspaper advertisements and her later letter to Clare – it is the gaps and corrections which are most telling. The silences, the "shadowy ambience" within Dinah's language, and her aggression towards the text, speak more powerfully than words the ghosts of her past, and point up the crypts of her traumatic memory. Gabriele Schwab notes that unspoken secrets can be seen to slowly destroy "the continuity of psychic life":

> Lives become shadow lives, simulacra of a hollowed-out normality. In this way, the buried ghosts of the past come to haunt language from within, always threatening to destroy its communicative and expressive function.
>
> Attacks on language are the material manifestations of attacks on memory, and yet it is language that preserves traces of the destroyed memory: this is the paradox of writings from the crypt. [43]

[43] Gabriele Schwab, "Writing Against Memory and Forgetting", *Literature and Medicine*, XXV/1 (Spring 2006), 103.

Through the "breakdown in language" prevalent in Bowen's later fiction, *The Little Girls* seeks to demonstrate the spectral power of traumatic memory to infiltrate the present.[44] Language itself becomes a crypt, each word enclosing, haunted by, unfolding repetitions of latent meaning.

The Little Girls thinks through the ways in which the crypt enables us to consider how the structures of traumatic memory and of literature shed light on each other. Bringing contemporary critical thought on cryptomimesis into dialogue with *The Little Girls* allows us to evaluate the interactions of time and identity in narrative, as well as the ways in which we might think about secrecy in literature in terms of a surface-depth model. These ideas have also enabled an examination of what this novel has to say about the repression of trauma and its manifestation in language, as well as the ways such disruptions to linear temporality might be represented in narrative. The present of *The Little Girls* is structurally and textually haunted by the secrets and promises of the past, suggesting that literature, the "ideal literary object", is best thought about as a combination of surface and depth, of secrecy and visibility, of text and shadow. Unpacking the cryptic and cryptomimetic structures set up by *The Little Girls* not only sheds light on this novel, but also provokes an unsettling of our thinking about the crypt itself, and indeed, about how we can and do read literature.

---

[44] Lee, *Elizabeth Bowen*, 197.

CHAPTER 9

HOWEVER: *EVA TROUT, OR CHANGING SCENES*

> The future, as we know, will resemble the past in being the result, largely, of a concatenation of circumstances. Many of our best moments, as well as our worst, are fortuitous. (*ET* 301)

> The truth, what I always have difficulty getting used to: that non-telepathy is possible. Always difficult to imagine that one can think something to oneself [*à part soi*], deep down inside, without being surprised by the other, without the other being immediately informed, as easily as if it had a giant screen in it, at the time of the talkies, with the remote control [*télécommande*] for changing channels and fiddling with the colours, the speech dubbed with large letters in order to avoid any misunderstanding. For foreigners and deaf-mutes .... Difficult to imagine a theory of what they still call the unconscious without a theory of telepathy.[1]

"However": simultaneously "deadly", "hopeless", "shutting-off", as Iseult Arble describes it, and yet unfinished, dragging with it the ghost of an ellipsis, an open space of continuation (*ET* 64). This single word, this word that causes Iseult – that causes the text – such distress, makes manifest the trauma work of this novel. The "however" of Eva is a "slippery fish" (*ibid.*, 213). In *Eva Trout, or Changing Scenes*, what was to be her final novel, Bowen disrupts all that has come before: "the scene", Austin asserts, "has indeed changed".[2] Eva's repeated and "misbegotten" (*ET* 64) "however" provokes logical and temporal disorientations, as *Eva Trout* and Eva Trout audaciously mimic and manipulate the "hopeless", thought-dead past: "Eva went

---

[1] Jacques Derrida, "Telepathy", trans. Nicholas Royle, *Oxford Literary Review*, X/1-2 (July 1988), 13-14.
[2] Austin, *Elizabeth Bowen*, 87.

to the dead clock, prised its glass face open and stood moving the hands round to imaginary hours" (*ibid.*, 149). *Eva Trout* simultaneously makes possible the future while utterly refusing it in a violently unambiguous, unchanging final scene. This is the conclusive set-piece to a narrative formed by changing screens and stills, from the castle which looks "as though cut out, flat, from a sheet of cardboard" (*ibid.*, 5), and its rooms which "began in a cardboard way to belong to history" (*ibid.*, 53); to Constantine, who seems as if he is a "figure cut from some picture but now pasted on to a blank screen" (*ibid.*, 40-41); as well as the two-dimensional representations of humanity in the National Portrait Gallery, all "pictures" and "images" (*ibid.*, 216); and the television screen which nightly sits "flickering [Eva and Jeremy] to sleep" (*ibid.*, 208). The novel shuffles each scene into place, presenting a new logic of screening the narrative. Such screens, with their subtitles for "foreigners and deaf-mutes", Derrida tells us, are analogous to the process of telepathy, practising unconscious communicative clarity and displaying thought.[3] To screen, however, is not only to show, but to hide. The changing stills, screens and scenes of *Eva Trout*, then, point up the processes not only inherent in telepathy, but also in lying; and in the sense that the psyche hides or lies about the presence of trauma, the novel's changing scenes also condition traumatic memory.

Eva's mishandling of "however" throughout the text foreshadows her son, Jeremy's, mishandling of the revolver at the novel's end, for both set in motion an expectation of the future, while underscoring its "deadly" uncertainty. Syntactical breaches in Eva's speech enact Derrida's declaration that "I posthume as I breathe", as the language of Eva Trout and of *Eva Trout* propels us towards the moment of death for the heroine and for the narrative. Yet even while Eva's corpse lies still warm, her life may be said to continue in Jeremy, in a Derridean act of "posthuming", of immortalization, which makes what Cixous calls "liars of life and death".[4] Eva's "dead body" (*ET* 109) weights the final sentence of Bowen's final novel, immovable and insurmountable, while she lies, still, interred within the silent tomb of Jeremy, who "was to be everything I shall not be", and who will

---

[3] Derrida, "Telepathy", 14.

[4] Jacques Derrida, *Jacques Derrida*, trans. Geoffrey Bennington, Chicago, IL: University of Chicago Press, 1993, 26; Cixous, *Portrait of Jacques Derrida*, 58.

survive her: he is the child, the issue, who shall carry on her name (*ibid.*, 220).

At the heart of the novel lies a lie: from where (and from whom) did Jeremy appear? *Eva Trout* locks away such secrets and its unspoken traumas – lies are elaborately constructed to hide these truths, to screen them from discovery. Like its characters, the novel hypnotizes, working to persuade or divert the reader away from these crypts, to swallow, instead, its lies. In reading *Eva Trout*, not only is one required to contend with the artificiality of a fictional narrative, and with the gaps and lacunae inherent in traumatic memory, but to remain aware – to keep in mind, or to remind oneself – of Eva Trout's and of *Eva Trout*'s anacolutha, their breaches of grammatical sequence. Eva's anacolutha figure the disruptive properties of the writing of trauma. That is, they call into question the ethics of narrative and its claim to realist representation as the anacoluthic lie reminds the reader that the novel one voraciously swallows is a fiction, and that what one had taken for fact is uncertain. This is the kind of "recognition of the danger inherent in all fiction-making" which Harriet Chessman asserts is at work across Bowen's fiction; "Stories are", she says, "quite simply, untrue; they capture us … in their nets".[5] In *Eva Trout*, even life and death are shown to be liars. In this chapter, I want to consider how a Derridean consideration of telepathy reveals how *Eva Trout* encourages the reader to "sense" when, to borrow a recurring pun of the novel, something "fishy" is going on, and moreover, what this kind of mind-reading might have to do with the writing of trauma.

Eva Trout is divided into two sections: the first, "Genesis", takes place in the months preceding and shortly after Eva comes into her inheritance, at the age of twenty-five; the second, "Eight Years Later", sees her return to England with her eight-year-old son, Jeremy. Eva was orphaned young: her mother, Cissie, died in an aeroplane crash while attempting to elope when Eva was an infant; her father, Willy, a wealthy businessman, committed suicide in Eva's adolescence. Since then, Eva has been left in the legal care of a "wicked guardian" (*ET* 72), her father's former lover, Constantine Ormeau. "Genesis" begins with Eva's departure from Larkins, the home of Iseult and Eric Arble,

---

[5] Harriet S. Chessman, "Women and Language in the Fiction of Elizabeth Bowen", *Twentieth-Century Literature*, XXIX (Spring 1983), 69.

for reasons never made quite clear except that, she says, "I cannot stay much longer where I now am" (*ibid.*, 25). She takes possession of a large house in Broadstairs and fills it with electrical appliances – "examples of everything auro-visual on the market this year" (*ibid.*, 124) – before she breaks the news to Iseult that she is "having a little child", and leads the elder woman to believe that the infant has been fathered by her own husband, Eric (*ibid.*, 128). The narrative propels forward six months; now in the United States, Eva mysteriously adopts not an illegitimate, but rather an illegal child.[6]

Eight years later, Eva returns to England accompanied by this child, Jeremy. Eva proposes marriage to her old friend, Henry Dancey, and although Henry initially refuses her, he does agree to stage a sham wedding departure at Victoria station, before once again changing his mind at the climactic moment and declaring Eva "My love, my sister" (*ibid.*, 297).[7] In the novel's final moments, just as the couple are about to set off, Jeremy dashes towards Eva holding a revolver which, wrapped in brown paper and string, and in a continuation of the post of *A World of Love*, has been passed from pillar to post throughout the novel, and shoots his mother dead. In its juxtaposition of death and life, of the heavy, still warmth of Eva's "dead body" (Bowen's last words, as it were) and of Jeremy, who "could not stop running on", this final (un)changing scene simultaneously forecloses the idea of a future and implies the possibility of immortality, of endless movement, helplessly propelled in a perpetual cycle of time and of thought, in which, "we know" (*ibid.*, 301), both past and future arise from an inextricable "concatenation of circumstances" (*ibid.*, 302).

However: in Eva's vocabulary this word is "pompous, it's unnatural-sounding, it's wooden, it's deadly, it's hopeless, it's shutting-off – the way *you* use it! it's misbegotten!" (*ibid.*, 64; original emphasis). That is, Eva fails to use "however" as a logical conjunction, as a link to a following (if contradictory) idea. "However" leads one to expect: it hangs with bated breath. Yet Eva's "however" is "deadly", it "shut[s]-off" our expectation of continuing

---

[6] The appearance of the child is anticipated at the beginning of the chapter by the inclusion of the Christmas carol "Silent Night", where ellipses do the work of the lines "round yon virgin, mother and child" (*ET* 139).

[7] There is a slippage here between Henry's love for Eva and for his dead sister, Louise, "my familiar" (*ibid.*, 165).

speech, the connection of one thought to another that Iseult describes (*ibid.*, 61). The "however" of *Eva Trout* and of Eva Trout is at once expectant and fallow (like, indeed, Eva herself), at once both and neither. "However" says and does two things at once. It is as if, notes Claire Connolly, the novel's syntax is "afraid to settle into fluency or to make itself at home in language".[8] Eva's mishandling of "however" foreshadows Jeremy's mishandling of the revolver at the novel's end – his own "however" to Eva's narrative – for both, while "deadly", also set in motion an expectation of the future, the desire to know, that is, what happens next.

This notion of an uncertain future is introduced in the novel's opening scene, when the Dancey children consider the limits of Eva's presence. Here, "however" carries across and brackets two sentences, while the tentative "perhaps" and the ellipses which follow the thought reinforce her indecision: "*How* long, they wondered, would this go on for? For ever and *ever*? Perhaps not …" (*ET* 4; my emphasis). *Eva Trout* frustrates this readerly longing for narrative continuity, for all of the events of the novel involve coming in after the fact, as it were, so that the reader never witnesses, for example, why Eva and the Arbles no longer see eye-to-eye, the breakdown of Iseult and Eric's marriage, or Eva's adoption of Jeremy. Indeed, like so much of the novel's correspondence, it seems as if we are always arriving, always "changing scenes", a moment too late. True narrative omniscience is refused in *Eva Trout*, and in this way carries on from the style and secrecy of *The Little Girls*. Moreover, this novel might be seen as a "however" to Bowen's body of work that refuses our desire for a final conclusive statement, while simultaneously deconstructing and destabilizing all that precedes it, or as Bennett and Royle state: "*Eva Trout* can thus be seen as a conclusion and a convulsion of the entire Bowen *oeuvre*."[9] These fluctuations are also present in the novel's ideas about identity, for its instability is, Corcoran notes, "sometimes so underminingly severe as to make the

---

[8] Claire Connolly, "(Be)Longing: The Strange Place of Elizabeth Bowen's *Eva Trout*", in *Borderlands: Negotiating Boundaries in Post-Colonial Writing*. ed. Monika Reif-Hülser, Amsterdam: Rodopi, 1999, 137.

[9] Bennett and Royle, *Elizabeth Bowen and the Dissolution of the Novel*, 143. See also Corcoran, *The Enforced Return*, 135; and Sinéad Mooney, "Unstable Compounds: Bowen's Beckettian Affinities", *Modern Fiction Studies*, LII/3 (Summer 2007), 251.

novel's modes of characterization congruent with radical postmodern conceptions of the hollowing-out of subjectivity, as characters – and Eva herself in particular – are virtually devoid of all continuity, becoming sites traversed by endless mobilities of desire".[10] It is this very discontinuity and perpetual desire that "however" enacts in *Eva Trout*, and which draws out the fracturing and the melancholic yearning which characterizes the memory of trauma.

In the sense that these instabilities of identity (Eva is "Constant in nothing" [*ET* 107]) and of "however" undermine the (grammatical) ethics of narrative, Eva's language might be described as criminal, according to Iseult's warning that she "shall fine you sixpence for each time you say 'however'" (*ibid.*, 64). Not only is Eva "wrong with the law" (*ibid.*, 166) (of the father, for her child has no father, or rather, she is his father, or her own father is her child's father), but she is wrong with the word, the patriarchal laws of language which Iseult, "the expert in English" (*ibid.*, 27), upholds.[11] Eva's language is thus outside the limits of correct or trustworthy speech. The misuse of the word "however" becomes a lie when it implies the qualification, continuation or justification of a point which never arrives, so that that in which the reader is led to believe never occurs. To read into the lacunae which haunt "however" is to put into practice a form of textual telepathy, an unwritten and unspoken exchange between author and reader which is nevertheless loaded with meaning. "However", in other words, replicates and sets in motion the significant themes of the novel and of Bowen's late fiction: lies, telepathy and the interactions of reading and writing.

"I never go back"

The novel posits in Eva and Iseult opposing temporal concerns; that is, while the younger woman more often looks to the future, Iseult is caught up in the past. Eva does not look back (*ibid.*, 60); twice, she explodes with incredulity at the very suggestion: "'*Back*'! – *I* never go *back*!" (*ibid.*, 17; original emphasis. See also 101). Hurt by Iseult's rejection of her love, Eva believes that the older woman "sent me back

[10] Corcoran, *The Enforced Return*, 128.

[11] Eva's sense of guilt regarding this trespass of the law is demonstrated by her reading of a passage of the "Gideon Bible" just prior to her receipt of Jeremy: "'*This is the law*,' she read" (*ET* 154; original emphasis).

… sent me back again – to be nothing" (*ibid.*, 203). Iseult, too, has watched Eva disappear into her propensity for "amnesia" (*ibid.*, 85): "Under this roof she's gone steadily back, back, back till of even the Eva there was there is not a trace" (*ibid.*, 95). The past for Eva, then, is synonymous with nothingness, vacuity, as Iseult recognizes when she states, "for her I'm over, I'm a thing of the past, and what's that to Eva?" (*ibid.*, 96). But Eva's suggestion that she record a conversation with Iseult is met with a flat refusal. For the latter, it is not posterity that is of interest, but the return of the past, and moreover, not only of looking back, but of hearing back: "How curious, yes, how very curious", Iseult remarks to Eva of her tape recorder, "if you'd had that thing years ago, when I knew you. What should we think of the playbacks, I do wonder?" The appeal of such a device lies, for Iseult, in its ability to represent the past just as it was, untainted by subjectivity, as she declares: "How I should like to play that scene over again: I should get a better grip on it next time" (*ibid.*, 126-27). Listening in, or eavesdropping on the past, a kind of belated understanding, is made possible by Eva's sophisticated instruments.[12]

Eva's instruments thus figure the temporal disruption and deferred action of the Freudian *Nachträglichkeit* – the sense, that is, that such a return would be "out of date" (*ibid.*, 245). Elsinore's return to the narrative, and to Eva's life, for example, is conditioned by this kind of belatedness. In fear of being "late by a minute" for her rendezvous with the child that will be Jeremy, Eva laments: "You came back too late, Elsinore. I cannot. You came at the wrong time." While Eva remains "Stopped at an intersection" – stilled at the crossroads of going back or "speed[ing]" forward – Elsinore and the past lose out to the future when the repressed, the "waiting thought", returns ("leap[s]") too late (*ibid.*, 154).[13] While for Iseult the tape recorder is an instrument concerned with the past, for Eva a recording is directed

[12] Eva's awareness of eavesdropping is clearest when she is expecting the telephone call regarding her child: "Going by, she shut the door of the bathroom, lest there be ears there" (*ibid.*, 154).

[13] Even Eva's future is capable of running late: a conversation "on the really rather momentous subject of Eva's future, had waited to get itself going till the last minute" (*ibid.*, 194). Iseult "had come too late on the scene" (*ibid.*, 10) to have any influence upon Eva's speech, Constantine resigns himself to being behind schedule, pointing out that "Late-comers can't be choosers" (*ibid.*, 108), and at the novel's conclusion, Eva worries that she has arrived too late (*ibid.*, 294).

towards the future: "It has recorded, 'Not on any account.' And it now records me saying, 'It has recorded, "Not on any account"'" (*ibid.*, 126). The dizzying prospect of an infinite regress of electronic recording implies continuity, a momentum of forward-looking (or forward-hearing), as well as the possibility of living-on, of the immortal encryption of Eva's voice, preserved for posterity. It echoes, hears again, the work of *The Little Girls*.

The repetition of trauma is enacted until the devastating finality of Eva's (and Bowen's) parting words on the platform of Victoria Station. Jeremy's "performance", or "game" played out in this closing scene is symbolic of the traumas – the losses, disappearances, misplacements and afterthoughts – by which it has been driven (*ibid.*, 298). *Eva Trout*, then, is an irrevocable game of *fort-da*, as described by Freud in *Beyond the Pleasure Principle*.[14] Caruth explains that this game

> … does not ultimately involve a symbolic representation of the mother's pleasurable return, but repeats, in a kind of stammer that interrupts its story, the painful memory of her departure …. What is most surprising in the child's game, however, is that this reenactment of reality in the game places repetition at the very heart of childhood, and links the repetition to a creative act of invention.[15]

In *Eva Trout*, the symbolic game is present in the stammering and amnesia which "overcome" Eva when only Eric visits her, and Iseult, the mother-figure does not: the latter fails to return after she has been rejected, cast away (*fort!*) by Eva (*ET* 85). The "creative act of invention" that Jeremy represents (in the sense that the story surrounding the child's procreation is a lie), might then be tied to the repetition of these traumatic departures (*da!*), as the news of Eva's forthcoming child is enough to drive Iseult away once again.

---

[14] In *Beyond the Pleasure Principle*, Freud describes watching his grandson throw a spool on a string from his cot and pulling it back over and over, calling "fort" ("gone") as he threw it and "da" ("here") as it returned. Freud interprets this as a reenactment of the traumatic departure and pleasurable return of the child's mother (see "Beyond the Pleasure Principle", 224-26).

[15] Cathy Caruth, "Parting Words: Trauma, Silence, and Survival", in *Acts of Narrative*, eds Carol Jacobs and Henry Sussman, Stanford, CA: Stanford University Press, 2003, 48.

These reverberations of maternal loss begin – for *Eva Trout*, at least – with the "unspeakable end" of Cissie Trout; they continue within the fraught relationship of Eva and Iseult; they haunt Eva's traumatic memory of her resistance to separation from Elsinore ("*Gone, gone …. Go away again.* WHAT ARE YOU DOING HERE?" [*ibid.*, 142; original emphasis]); and they finish, finally, with Jeremy's ironic vengeance, forcing permanent departure on the mother who proposes to desert him (*ibid.*, 34). The act of casting away and returning to the mother-figure, which has been described and enacted again and again in Bowen's work (perhaps most clearly in my discussions of *The Hotel* and *The House in Paris*, for example), is at its height in this last novel, where it reaches its terrible conclusion with the reunion of mother and child (*da*) occurring at the same time as the mother's departure (*fort*). The destruction of the mother at the moment of embrace both shatters and replicates the trauma which has repeatedly appeared in and conditioned Bowen's writing, bringing it to a theatrical climax before the curtain drops on the scene, on the novel, on Bowen's career and on Eva, who will "remain gone" (*fort*) (*ibid.*, 203). In the frieze of this final scene – a "stage, or platform" (*ibid.*, 298) from which no one departs – the reader is unable to part from death. Like Jeremy, the reader is presented with the dead weight of this maternal corpse, so that one cannot move for "fall[ing] over", as we stumble and stammer across the perpetuity of a trauma that will not die, that will survive itself, and that will live on posthumously (*ibid.*, 302).[16]

"What is 'concatenation'?"

Yet, in Eva's "misbegotten" "however", even the possibility of a future is a lie, for although it implies continuity, suggesting there is more to come, she fears that "at the end of it all you'll find out that I have nothing to declare" (*ET* 64). Indeed, "at the end of it all", she does not "declare", but rather queries. Her final words, "Constantine … what is 'concatenation'?" not only make clear Eva's inability to

[16] Corcoran also notes this impossibility of surmounting Eva, the dead mother, and points out that Jeremy "is, of course, with a terrible irony, sealing his own fate as one final orphaned child in the work of Elizabeth Bowen" (*The Enforced Return*, 136). In fact, it is ultimately Eva, rather than Jeremy, who is "an obstacle not to be overcome" (*ET* 222).

understand "concatenation", but to put it into practice, for these "last words" represent a perpetually unanswered doubt which opposes the concatenation of thought (*ibid.*, 301). Moreover, it is not Eva who ultimately enacts an absence of speech, but Constantine: "I have nothing to say. Nothing to declare. No statement" (*ibid.*, 296).[17] The phrase "No statement" suggests, if not an outright falsehood, then a reluctance to speak the truth, neither confirmation nor denial, thereby performing an evasion similar to Eva's "manner of speaking … like a displaced person". But, if it is true that Eva "had nothing *to* say that could not be said, adequately, the way she said it", so that whatever she does say cannot be pinned down, cannot be concatenated, it might be that all Eva has to say is a lie (*ibid.*, 10; original emphasis). Conspiracy is, after all, "the air natural to her" (*ibid.*, 96); indeed, what part of such a claim as "I am a liar …. I am not always" (*ibid.*, 248), can one believe? An amnesiac's words are always already "dubious", as Sinéad Mooney points out: "The amnesiac subject, all sure grasp of the past dissolving, has the dubious freedom to rearrange ad nauseam the elements of a posited selfhood into some new form, the self becoming an endless series of such refashionings, or nobody at all, the fear that is behind Eva's endless spinning of lies, fictions, and fantasies."[18] In this way, memory becomes bound up with questions of truth and of deception, and moreover, of the ethics of fictional narrative.

Derrida asserts that "like the self-identity of the subject, memory *is* or rather *must*, *should* be an ethical obligation: infinite and at every instant" – indeed, memory must survive, it must live on, still.[19] Eva's memory is inconstant, and her identity, as I have discussed, is unstable, almost anticipating Derrida's suggestion that the "essential finitude of a discontinuous anamnesis inscribes ellipses and eclipses in the identity of the subject".[20] Her failure to meet Derrida's ethical demand and moreover, the failure of the novel itself to do so – for

---

[17] "Nothing *is* final, I suppose", says Constantine, in a frustratingly indecisive, indefinite turn of phrase (*ET* 296; original emphasis). Further, both Eva and Constantine appear to have inherited or borrowed this trait of having "nothing to declare" from Willy Trout, whose suicide "left nothing more to be said" (*ibid.*, 96).

[18] Mooney, "Unstable Compounds", 253.

[19] Jacques Derrida, "'Le Parjure', *Perhaps*: Storytelling and Lying ('Abrupt Breaches of Syntax')", in Jacobs and Sussman, *Acts of Narrative*, 197 (original emphasis).

[20] *Ibid.*, 201.

such instabilities necessarily transfer to the eponymous title, a title shakily supported by its precarious subtitle, "changing scenes" – reminds us, once again, of the lies which permeate the text. It is as if one is thrust into the midst of "the malicious lying of [Eva's] misleading dreams in which she was no one, nowhere" (*ET* 50), dreams that Eva even denies having: "You had curious dreams", Constantine remarks; "I did not", Eva replies (*ibid.*, 108). The power of dreams and of narrative to be misleading can occur in three ways, as identified by Miller in the context of a discussion of Marcel Proust. Miller argues that the misleading power of narrative has to do "with storytelling (in the double sense of lying and of narration), with memory as a precarious support of narrative continuity, and with anacoluthon's function in both storytelling and lying".[21] In reading *Eva Trout*, not only is one required to contend with the artificiality of a fictional narrative, and with the gaps and lacunae inherent in traumatic memory, but to remain aware – to keep in mind, or to remind oneself – of the novel's, and of Eva's, anacolutha. Only in *Eva Trout*, in Eva's "however", do such transgressions against language also become a crime committed against the text. The implied future of the misuse of "however", discovered to be a lie, calls into question the novel's internal realism.

To put it another way: the two greatest hoaxes or fictions of the novel are Eva's maternity and her marriage, so that she performs, thereby, the construction of her gender identity. Jeremy, Bennett and Royle point out, "is a simulacrum of a son", while the final fictional departure of the bridal tour "draws together the text's theorization of fictionality, its dissolution of the novel .... The entire scene is undecidably a *staged* event".[22] Any prop for this last scene, the novel points out, "could have been a fake" (*ET* 300). All is designed, for this performance, to "[look] more lifelike" (*ibid.*, 300), although "no life was more real than this" (*ibid.*, 216). Realism, though it maintains a pretence to the real is, of course, a work of fiction, always a lie. Derrida confesses that he prefers the word "invention" to "lie", precisely because

[21] J. Hillis Miller, *Reading Narrative*, Norman: University of Oklahoma Press, 1998, 149.

[22] Bennett and Royle, *Elizabeth Bowen and the Dissolution of the Novel*, 141, 155 (original emphasis).

> … it *hesitates perhaps* between *creative* invention, the production of what is not – or was not earlier – and *revelatory* invention, the discovery and unveiling of what *already* is or finds itself to be there. Such an invention thus hesitates *perhaps*, it is suspended undecidably between fiction and truth, but also between lying and veracity, that is, between perjury and fidelity.[23]

I have pointed out that Jeremy is a (pro)creative invention; Eva's marriage, moreover, is an example of revelatory invention, thought to be a hoax but finally revealed as "true" love. Eva herself, then, "hesitates *perhaps*" between these two pillars of invention, her identity "suspended undecidably between" the illegality or "perjury" of her maternity and the "fidelity" of her matrimony; perched, indeed, on the liminality of her "however".

Eva Trout (like Eric) is recidivist – through its lies and textual transgressions it relapses into the offences of *The Little Girls*. These crimes are at times literal – as, for example, when Jeremy is kidnapped by Iseult, and is earlier acquired rather shadily by Eva – or psychological, as when Eva suspects Iseult's identity to have been stolen: "Had this *been* Miss Smith, or was she dead and somebody impersonating her?" (*ibid.*, 212; original emphasis). Iseult behaves like a criminal, purposefully masking her identity, the scar that would betray her:

> The hair was dark, but worn in a bull fringe coming low down … so that one could not see what was underneath. One was not meant to? It was as though to hide something, some disfigurement, scar or burn or a birth-mark. (*Ibid.*, 218-19)

By hiding the identifying mark and by refusing to pin down what such a blemish might be ("some disfigurement, scar or burn or a birth-mark"), by both concealing and misrepresenting, both Iseult and the novel resist verisimilitude.[24] Just as Iseult hides the revolver, her

---

[23] Derrida, "Le Parjure", 202 (original emphasis).

[24] The difference between the two types of lies is made clear by Dr Bonnard: "[Jeremy] has not yet incurred the ability to lie. We must remember, he is on the eve of doing so …. So far, he has been able to conceal, not yet, however, to misrepresent" (*ET* 249). Being "on the *eve* of doing so", suggests that he may learn this ability from his mother, Eva.

illegal weapon, in the crypt-like boxes of Eva's property, falsely claiming that it belongs to the younger woman with the defiant assertion that "It's no business of theirs what is inside", the novel embeds the possibility of a deadly truth within a fictional narrative (*ibid.*, 252). The novel's lies deny omniscience and protect what it is "no business" of ours to know. Realism is revealed to be fraudulent: "Hoaxed, were they? An unreal act collects round it real-er emotion than a real act, sometimes, [Henry] thought" (*ibid.*, 293).

Realist fiction, then, performs a confidence trick on the reader by imbuing this "unreal act" with "real-er emotion". Constantine's written words do this, Iseult recognizes:

> … what a way to write, what garlands of affectation! Yet, to give him credit, this was quite a performance. This mannered manner of his was not quite the thing; no. Yet the ambiguities had one sort of merit, or promise – one was at least on the verge of the Henry James country. (*Ibid.*, 27-28)

This writing, however, merely performs the "promise", as Constantine's "affectation" of literature only shadows what Iseult sees as the real writing of James. This is not the only letter given word-for-word in the text – letters, postcards, telegrams (and the "ghastly parcel" that is the revolver, carefully wrapped in brown paper and string [*ibid.*, 252]) are delivered back and forth throughout. The form and content of the novel thus enact the hypnotic power of story-telling, designed to convince the reader to believe in the truth or reality of this fiction, this "unreal act".

Mr Dancey, for example, whose novel is not yet complete, is perpetually caught in the redrafting of his written words, trying to capture his fictional world in its entirety but suffering for the realism of his art:

> You remember he once was writing a book? Well, he still is. Every now and then, he comes up against something which makes him have to go right back and re-cast the whole thing from the beginning. (*Ibid.*, 262)[25]

[25] Elsinore behaves similarly: she "wrote and re-wrote the same long letter, which she read aloud, then tore up, then began again" (*ET* 50).

He is still writing, writing still, for his task is futile, Iseult gravely asserts: "Life is an anti-novel" (*ibid.*, 228). True realism is impossible, for we can never know the "whole story", especially in a novel which insists upon delivering us to the destinations of its plot too late: "If you'd ever been more than partially honest with me, if you'd ever given me anything like the whole picture, or whole story .... But perhaps there is no whole picture, or story", Iseult writes in a letter to Constantine (*ibid.*, 229). Indeed, "perhaps", there is not: an ambiguous admission which finally speaks the truth. Eva, the amnesiac, is unable to "reassemble the picture", to know the whole story, and so, neither can her reader. In this way, the text figures the problems of a memory shattered by death and trauma. When even writing within the novel is gestated under the weight of the memorial of the dead, it is hardly surprising that life, or the "real", is difficult to maintain, that Iseult's novel "was born dead" (*ibid.*, 253), and that we are ultimately faced with the dead weight of Eva Trout's and *Eva Trout*'s corpse; that is, with a writing of trauma. Yet *Eva Trout* survives, it posthumes, immortal, defying the death of textuality.

Ghost writing and mind reading

Such "ghost writing", as we might call it, draws on notions of telepathy, "a concept and effect intimately bound up with writing and death, the spectral and unprogrammable".[26] Henry's discovery of a verse written by his dead sister, Louise, in the flyleaf of her prayer-book, is not only a figure of prosopopeia, a letter or medium that crosses that "thin" wall "Between [the] dead and [the] living", but as an immortal and telepathic communication between past and present (*ET* 190). Reading the writing of the past "restored to Henry, for some reason, not so much Louise as the original savagery of loss" (*ibid.*, 281); such textual telepathy is more concerned with the return of (the repressed) "real-er emotion" than it is with a conjuring of spirits. In a mind reading of *Eva Trout*, then, telepathy begins to unravel or to build upon ideas about memory, especially the memory of trauma. Jeremy's "extra-sensory" communication with Eva forms another repetition of his *fort-da* game present, Derrida observes, in the very word, "telepathy":

---

[26] Nicholas Royle, "The 'Telepathy Effect': Notes Toward a Reconsideration of Narrative Fiction", in Jacobs and Sussman, *Acts of Narrative*, 109.

> *Fort: Da, tele*pathy against tele*pathy*, distance against menacing immediacy, but also the opposite, feeling [*le sentiment*] (always close to oneself, it is thought), against the suffering of distancing [*la souffrance de l'éloignment*] that would also be called telepathy.[27]

Eva and Jeremy's telepathy, then, simultaneously sympathetically joins them (*da*) and recalls the physical distance between them (*fort*), just as their final embrace both unites and destroys their bond. That dramatic conclusion seems predestined or predicted by narrative clairvoyance, by the description of Eva as "gun shy" (*ET* 81), the small children playing with guns in the background of the Christmas-shopping scene (*ibid.*, 140), and the "pocket-size toy revolver" Jeremy chooses as a present from Iseult (*ibid.*, 274).[28] Moreover, Henry appears to see Eva herself as clairvoyant when he asks her, "What's supposed to be going to happen, Eva?" – to which her monosyllabic and illogical reply is "Why?" (*ibid.*, 260). The instabilities of question and answer here repeat the uncertain future of Eva's "however", and the "Why, however?" of her response to Iseult's explanation of the process of thought (*ibid.*, 61). Why should one think, or think of the future, into the future, Eva asks, while the reader's knowledge that she has no future beyond the text gives her words the eerie resonance of the speech of the dead.

Jeremy's powers of seeing make him a formidable reader of and in the text; he is able to "[look] more deeply into … images than [Eva] did. Torn skies, curdled waters, hieroglyphic smoke he had had a particular way of scanning" (*ibid.*, 207), while his mother cannot even read the familiarity of her own hand: "Extending the palm of her right hand to be read by the flames, she leaned over the fate-lines in it uncomprehendingly" (*ibid.*, 100).[29] Indeed, Eva is at one time frightened to begin reading (*ET* 59). This betrays her amnesia: unable or unwilling to read a text, she similarly avoids an active examination

---

[27] Derrida, "Telepathy", 36 (original emphasis).

[28] Fate and destiny circumscribe *Eva Trout* – "fate magnetizes all of us" (*ET* 269): Iseult "seemed destined to have Eva" (*ibid.*, 9); Portman believes his meeting with Eva to be due to "the hand of fate" or "the mathematical probabilities of chance" (*ibid.*, 131); and Eva worries that in encouraging Jeremy to overcome his disability, she has "diverted" his destiny (*ibid.*, 260).

[29] Bennett and Royle term Jeremy a figure of reading (*Elizabeth Bowen and the Dissolution of the Novel*, 143).

of the past. But Iseult reads too much: "I have lived through books. I have lived internally" (*ibid.*, 96). Iseult has sustained herself, she has survived on and through writing, lived on and through stories – indeed, on and through Eva's lies. In a different context, Mary Jacobus points out the parallels between reading and incorporation or consumption, so that we might describe Iseult as a "voracious reader".[30] If it is true that reading "is actually a method of taking someone else's thoughts inside oneself", or "a way of eating another person's words", then Iseult swallows more lies than any other character of *Eva Trout*, too ready to believe others when they are telling stories.[31] Iseult might do better to direct at herself her admonishing question to Constantine, "don't you think you've been reading too many stories?" (*ET* 231-32). To be sure, books "are not … to be simply gazed at", but by the same token, they are not to be swallowed whole or taken on face value (*ibid.*, 59). It is fiction's task to hypnotize the reader into believing its stories, to persuade us of the truth of its lies. Iseult, however, is an uncritical reader of the fiction of *Eva Trout* and Eva Trout: this malleable subject is too obsessed by Eva to see outside the covers of her fiction – that is "the whole of the picture" (*ibid.*, 254).

In this respect, fiction, the novel, parallels the performance of traumatic memory: both are defined by the appearance, or act of verisimilitude, when in truth, they are but a lie: "Nothing hidden except what was in the books" (*ibid.*, 60). Indeed, the very function of traumatic memory is to protect consciousness from the truth of the sorrow it encrypts, to keep even the secret of the trauma's existence. In one way, this necessitates lying to oneself – and believing it – describing the critical division between what we might call "healthy" memory, and traumatic memory, so that the interaction of thought between these two states, still present within one mind, is made impossible. To return to Derrida's statement, to the "difficulty" with which I began this chapter, traumatic memory becomes concerned with the distances constructed within the psyche, and with the ability of a separated consciousness to communicate across its traumatic partitions. How is it that "one can think something to oneself … deep

---

[30] Mary Jacobus, *Psychoanalysis and the Scene of Reading*, Oxford: Oxford University Press, 1999, 20.

[31] Alix Strachey, "Some Unconscious Factors in Reading" (1930), cited in *ibid.*, 29.

down inside, without being surprised by the other"? How does the conscious mind remain unaware of the crypt, and how does its guardian protect the secret of trauma?

In his study of literature and telepathy, Royle makes use of the term "cryptaesthesia" which, he explains, etymologically "pertains to the perception (*aesthesis*) of what is hidden (*crypto-*)".[32] The protective lies and distances of traumatic memory could be overcome by the practice of cryptaesthesia, the ability to sense that something is hidden and perhaps, to recover it. In this way, the cryptaesthesia of *Eva Trout* works to resurrect the traumatic memories of *The Little Girls*. This is most clearly seen in the return of the repressed revolver to the narrative, and the repetitions of its burial and revival. Iseult searches for a site in which to inter the gun – requesting that Constantine keep it locked in his safe, before leaving it as an anonymous parcel among Eva's belongings (*ET* 251). Jeremy, however, digs it up, immediately sensing the presence of the carton or crypt, and determined to unearth the revolver – "He did not require to dig deep; something immediately met his hands. The parcel was as weighty as it was curious; he bore it back with him to the sofa, where he sawed away at the heavily-knotted string with his little pocket-knife" (*ibid.*, 287-88) – before reluctantly stowing it away once again in a drawer beneath a pile of gloves, recalling this same hiding-place from *The Little Girls*.

In a similar way, and like Leopold in *The House in Paris* or Jane in *A World of Love*, Jeremy seeks to rummage through Iseult's mind: "Don't imagine he for a moment cared for me, but for that one flash – I was a walking strong-box he wanted to rifle" (*ibid.*, 274). Indeed, her very words contain the revolver ("rifle") and crypt ("strong-box"). Jeremy wastes his time on Iseult, however, for she has "undergone an emotional hysterotomy, and am the better" – since her (pro)creation, a novel, was "born dead", her "inside's gone" (*ibid.*, 251). It is not "nothing" that Iseult hides (she does, after all, disguise her face with a fringe), but it is at the same time *nothing*: the trauma of her emptiness and inability to produce even a fiction-child – either a novel, or an

---

[32] The word "cryptaesthesia" was coined by Charlies Richet in the late-nineteenth century and is defined in the *OED* as "A supernormal faculty of perception, whether clairvoyant or telepathic" (see Nicholas Royle, *Telepathy and Literature: Essays on the Reading Mind*, Oxford: Basil Blackwell, 1991, 60).

infant born from a lie. A cryptaesthetic reading of *Eva Trout*, then, points up the perception of these lies and lacunae in the text, and through the novel's concern with telepathy, leads us to sense its memory of trauma, the trauma of a certain nothing.

Eva's dead body

> All-in-all, what a literature – of what? Longing. The lyricism of forgetfulness. The nightmare of the frustrated passion. (*Ibid.*, 119)

Bowen's writing works towards the terrible conclusion of this last novel, its agony of "Longing", "forgetfulness" and "frustrated passion" that is finally attempted to be laid to rest in Eva's corpse. "Still, you'd prefer me dead", Eva asserts, "Silent forever, in my tomb"; indeed, her doom is to lie still, and to lie, still, interred within the silent tomb of Jeremy (*ibid.*, 109). The novel's final words, its conclusive scene of Eva's "dead body", are *Eva Trout*'s final "however": deathly still, Eva Trout ends while *Eva Trout* goes on. The novel thus survives the protagonist it endlessly revives for future readers, since in Bowen's corpus, "More has been buried than you know" (*ibid.*, 111).

Postscript

> "Still, you ought to get going."
> "Going?" he asked warily, with a frown.
> "To wherever it is. To somewhere else."
> "That is not so simple," he said, "as you seem to think." (*PC* 72)

> I posthume as I breathe.[1]

When Bowen died in 1973, she left, along with the partial draft of an autobiography, the first chapter of a novel, to be titled "The Move-In". Her literary executor published these with other collected writings posthumously as *Pictures and Conversations* (1974). This title, taken from the opening sentence of Lewis Carroll's work, *Alice in Wonderland* (1865),[2] Spencer Curtis Brown notes, "was significant, for the book would never have dealt with her own adult life, but only with images that her eyes had seen and with memories of things said to her".[3] Bowen's autobiography, then, was not planned as a factual or historical rendering of her life, but as a work of memory, a personal work of subjectivity. In this final work coheres Bowen's career-long concern with memorializing the past. But in this conclusion I do not want to depart from my discussion of Bowen's fiction towards a consideration of her autobiographical fragments. Rather, I want to think about the ways in which "The Move-In", Bowen's fictional remains and a text neglected by critical appraisal, draws out the concerns of trauma and writing present throughout Bowen's *oeuvre*, and develops these in the context of the posthumous voice. If it is true,

[1] Derrida, *Jacques Derrida*, 26.
[2] "Alice was beginning to get very tired of sitting by her sister on the bank, and of having nothing to do: once or twice she had peeped into the book her sister was reading, but it had no pictures or conversations in it, 'and what is the use of a book,' thought Alice, 'without pictures or conversations?'" (Lewis Carroll, *"Alice's Adventures in Wonderland" and "Through the Looking-Glass, and What Alice Found There"* (1865), Oxford: Oxford University Press, 2008, 9).
[3] Brown, "Foreword", viii.

as I have argued in the last chapter, that the conclusion of *Eva Trout* constitutes a stammering perpetuation of trauma and of death beyond which the text does not – indeed, cannot – progress, then it follows that "The Move-In" is a posthumous text not only in terms of the dead body of the author, and of Eva, her final heroine, but the dead body of her fiction. The fragment or ghost of "The Move-In" remains, disrupting the stilled corpus of Bowen's fictional *oeuvre*. This book has explored the ways in which Bowen's fiction complicates existing models of trauma theory in its exploration of the ethics of writing as survival, and has investigated the intersections of trauma and writing in Bowen's fictional work, with particular emphasis on the ways in which this gives rise to an understanding of memory and of secrecy in narrative. "The Move-In" works as a postscript to Bowen's fiction, a belated addition that calls attention to the characteristics of writing after death, of writing after trauma.

This novel fragment describes the arrival of three friends at what appears to be an Anglo-Irish Big House, expecting hospitality from the aunt of an acquaintance they have made while travelling. However, the house at which they have arrived is not the home of "Simon's" aunt. The group, out of fuel and out of money, resist the protestations of the woman who does live here, and at this first chapter's suspenseful conclusion, suggest that they stay in the house's ominously "uninhabited wing" (*PC* 76). Even in this short fragment, the text enacts a struggle between arrival and departure, between moving in and going away, between life and death, hovering like "a wisp of ectoplasm" called into being by a kind of novelistic "séance" (*PC* 68). Bowen's characteristic threshold conclusion here instead works as an introduction to the novel: the effect produced is of a narrative unable to decide where to go, whether or not to begin. Bowen's writing, in "The Move-In" and elsewhere is, as Cixous says of Carroll's,

> … a form of writing which doesn't settle in one place any more than a bird or an operation, but skips, flutters, moves, "out of breath," without trying to maintain sense or catch it, but moved by the curiosity – in the etymological sense of the word – which it feels

> about its own existence: the very writing questions itself about what it will possibly be able to say, what it's going to do, how far it's going.[4]

"Going?" This book has tried to show that in Bowen's work, this kind of breathless questioning of writing itself works as a traumatic deconstruction of its own function. Self-referential linguistic multiplicity and fracturing in Bowen's writing thus becomes at once a means of representing trauma in narrative, and a statement about the impossibility of doing so.

In "The Move-In", even as the novel's title promises entrance into the house, into the narrative, the text itself refuses and resists reading. It is conditioned by the impossibility of crossing a threshold. These visitors (and this text) are going nowhere. They audaciously unpack the boot of their car and strew their belongings (a miscellaneous array of items – a "lidless pot of ointment", "a half-eaten banana", a broken watch, a seagull's wing – packed away, it seems, since *The Little Girls*) across the gravel (*PC* 73). Their boot operates like Nicholas Royle's portmanteau, the "question" of which "is perhaps also that of the crypt".[5] Recalling the secrecy of the ideal literary object which, I have argued, is part of the project of *The Little Girls*, "The Move-In" works as a crypt for the earlier novel and, perhaps, for all of Bowen's fiction. Just as the crypt describes both the structure and the space within, "The Move-In" at once houses and constitutes the trauma of Bowen's writing. Like Cixous' breathless writing, "a kind of portmanteau writing" may be seen as a "familiar other name for deconstruction".[6] The boot or portmanteau of "The Move-In" thus becomes a model of the deconstructive work of Bowen's writing and, moreover, of the deconstructive work of the writing of trauma.

But "The Move-In" will not spill. It operates as an abortive fragment. The chapter's final words, "No – impossible!", the woman's refusal of her unexpected guests' desire to stay, come to signify absolute secrecy and a negation of narrative momentum (*PC* 76). Like the strangers' car, the novel has insufficient vitality, insufficient fuel,

---

[4] Hélène Cixous, "Introduction to Lewis Carroll's *Through the Looking-Glass* and *The Hunting of the Snark*", trans. Marie Maclean, *New Literary History*, XIII/2 (Spring 1982), 234.

[5] Nicholas Royle, "Portmanteau", *New Literary History*, XXXVII/1 (Winter 2006), 243.

[6] *Ibid.*, 241.

with which to go on. In spite of the precipitant movement of the novel's to-be title, the narrative chokes. Bowen, the car, the novel: out of breath. Impossible. If it is the case, then, that Bowen's writing may be seen to "[question] itself about what it will possibly be able to say, what it's going to do, how far it's going", that abrupt end to the fragment refuses to say or to do anything: the novel, like the visitors, will not go anywhere. Unfinished, "The Move-In" becomes a statement of its own impossibility, of its own death, of that traumatic secret which, finally, cannot be spoken, that which "escapes text".[7] It is a fitting and logical conclusion to Bowen's writing of trauma that her work should expire in silence.

In the final analysis, survival is the nature of Bowen's fiction; writing constitutes survival. "The Move-In" is the posthumous postscript to Bowen's writing of trauma, an afterthought, a half-thought. It is not only her wartime fiction that, as Marina MacKay has recognized, is characterized by "an ominous air of unfinished business", but rather, the whole body of her writing.[8] "The Move-In" is a novel that is only a beginning; like the maid seen through the windows of the house, it is "disembodied" (*PC* 68). And even as it calls attention to the traumatic characteristics of the posthumous text, torn off and inscribed by untranslatable death, "The Move-In" is a disembodied text, a ghostly posthumous narration by a disembodied voice that, going nowhere, insists upon its own survival.[9] "I posthume as I breathe", writes Derrida – may as well have been written by Bowen. And "There you have him then", asserts Cixous:

> … he who dies at the top of his lungs, a buried-alive supernatural, who gets wind of a new definition of immortality through the magic of writing. A frenzy of activity …. He writes as he posthumes. The writing is his survivor, she [*l'écriture, f.*] survives *him.*[10]

---

[7] "The portmanteau comes to designate the double logic of the 'escaping text' and what 'escapes text'" (Royle, "Portmanteau", 242).

[8] Marina MacKay, "World War II, the Welfare State, and Postwar 'Humanism'", in *The Cambridge Companion to the Twentieth-Century English Novel*, ed. Robert L. Caserio, Cambridge: Cambridge University Press, 148.

[9] See, for example, Claire Raymond, *The Posthumous Voice in Women's Writing from Mary Shelley to Sylvia Plath*, Aldershot: Ashgate, 2006, 221.

[10] Cixous, *Portrait of Jacques Derrida*, 58-59 (original emphasis).

Writing remains, it houses one's remains, it is one's remains. It makes "liars of life and death".[11] Bowen's writing is breathless writing, posthumous writing, deconstructive writing: Bowen's writing is the writing of trauma.

[11] *Ibid.*, 58.

Bibliography

References to items held in the Elizabeth Bowen Collection (TXRC98-A9) at the Harry Ransom Humanities Research Centre, University of Texas at Austin, are given as "HRHRC", followed by the box and file number.

Works by Elizabeth Bowen (in chronological order)

Bowen, Elizabeth, "The Back Drawing-Room" (1926), in Bowen, *Collected Stories*, 199-210.

—, *The Hotel* (1927), Harmondsworth: Penguin, 1987.

—, *The Last September* (1929), New York: Anchor Books, 2000.

—, *Friends and Relations* (1931), Harmondsworth: Penguin, 1943.

—, *To the North* (1932), London: Vintage, 1999.

—, "The Apple Tree" (1934), in Bowen, *Collected Stories*, 461-70.

—, "The Mulberry Tree" (1934), in Bowen, *The Mulberry Tree*, 13-21.

—, *The House in Paris* (1935), Harmondsworth: Penguin, 1976.

—, "Preface to *The Faber Book of Modern Short Stories*" (1936), in Bowen, *Collected Impressions*, 38-46.

—, *The Death of the Heart* (1938), New York: Anchor, 2000.

—, "The Big House" (1940), in Bowen, *The Mulberry Tree*, 25-30.

—, "The Demon Lover" (1941), in Bowen, *Collected Stories*, 661-66.

—, "A Love Story: 1939" (1941), in Bowen, *Collected Stories*, 497-511.

—, "Summer Night" (1941), in Bowen, *Collected Stories*, 583-608.

—, "Sunday Afternoon" (1941), in Bowen, *Collected Stories*, 616-22.

—, "Tears, Idle Tears" (1941), in Bowen, *Collected Stories*, 479-87.

—, *Seven Winters: Memories of a Dublin Childhood* (1942), London: Longmans, 1943.

—, *Bowen's Court* (1942), New York: Ecco, 1979.

—, "Notes on Eire", The National Archives, DO130/28, 1942 (as Elizabeth Cameron).

—, "The Happy Autumn Fields" (1944), in Bowen, *Collected Stories*, 671-85.

—, "The Inherited Clock" (1944), in Bowen, *Collected Stories*, 623-40.

—, "Mysterious Kôr" (1944), in Bowen, *Collected Stories*, 728-40.

—, "I Hear You Say So" (1945), in Bowen, *Collected Stories*, 751-57.
—, "Ivy Gripped the Steps" (1945), in Bowen, *Collected Stories*, 686-711.
—, "Postscript to *The Demon Lover*" (1945), in Bowen, *The Mulberry Tree*, 94-99.
—, "Out of a Book" (1946), in Bowen, *The Mulberry Tree*, 48-53.
—, "Preface to *Uncle Silas*, by Sheridan Le Fanu" (1947), in Bowen, *The Mulberry Tree*, 100-13.
—, Letter to Daniel George, 2 June 1948, HRHRC 10.4.
—, *The Heat of the Day* (1949), New York: Anchor, 2002.
—, "A Year I Remember: 1918", broadcast 10 March 1949, HRHRC 2.3.
—, "Outrageous Ladies" [1949-63], in Bowen, *People, Places, Things*, 379-83.
—, *Collected Impressions*, London: Longmans Green, 1950.
—, "Elizabeth Bowen and Jocelyn Brooke in Conversation", broadcast 3 October 1950, HRHRC 2.3.
—, "London, 1940" (1950), in Bowen, *The Mulberry Tree*, 21-25.
—, "The Bend Back" (1950), in Bowen, *The Mulberry Tree*, 54-60.
—, "The Cult of Nostalgia", broadcast 4 August 1951, HRHRC 2.3.
—, *The Shelbourne* (1951), London: Vintage, 2001.
—, "The Art of Respecting Boundaries" (1952), in Bowen, *People, Places, Things*, 397-400.
—, "Preface to *The Last September*" (1952), in Bowen, *The Mulberry Tree*, 122-26.
—, *A World of Love* (1954), New York: Anchor, 2003.
—, "Interview with John Bowen, William Craig, and W.N. Ewer", broadcast 11 September 1959, HRHRC 2.3.
—, "Preface to *Stories by Elizabeth Bowen*" (1959), in Bowen, *The Mulberry Tree*, 126-30.
—, *A Time in Rome* (1959), London: Vintage, 2003.
—, *Afterthought: Pieces About Writing*, London: Longmans, 1962.
—, "Sources of Influence" (1962), in Lassner, *Elizabeth Bowen: A Study of the Short Fiction*, 145-47.
—, *The Little Girls* (1963), New York: Anchor, 2004.
—, *The Good Tiger* (1965), London: Jonathan Cape, 1970.
—, *Eva Trout, or Changing Scenes* (1968), New York: Anchor, 2003.
—, *Pictures and Conversations*, London: Allen Lane, 1974.

—, *The Mulberry Tree: Writings of Elizabeth Bowen*, ed. Hermione Lee, San Diego, CA: Harcourt Brace Jovanovich, 1986.

—, *The Collected Stories of Elizabeth Bowen*, ed. Angus Wilson, London: Vintage, 1999.

—, *The Bazaar and Other Stories*, ed. Allan Hepburn, Edinburgh: Edinburgh University Press, 2008.

—, *People, Places, Things: Essays by Elizabeth Bowen*, ed. Allan Hepburn, Edinburgh: Edinburgh University Press, 2008.

—, Draft of "Preface to *The Last September*" (n.d.), HRHRC 7.2.

—, "Ireland" (n.d.), HRHRC 6.5.

—, Material for the *Broadsheet* (n.d.), HRHRC 1.5.

—, Notes for a public reading of *The Little Girls* (n.d.), HRHRC 7.4.

Secondary sources

Abraham, Nicolas, "Notes on the Phantom: A Complement to Freud's Metapsychology" (1975), in Abraham and Torok, *The Shell and the Kernel*, 171-76.

—, "The Shell and the Kernel", trans. Nicholas T. Rand, *Diacritics*, IX/1 (Spring 1979), 15-28.

Abraham, Nicolas, and Maria Torok, "'The Lost Object – Me': Notes on Endocryptic Identification" (1975), in Abraham and Torok, *The Shell and the Kernel*, 139-56.

—, "Mourning *or* Melancholia: Introjection *versus* Incorporation" (1972), in Abraham and Torok, *The Shell and the Kernel*, 125-38.

—, "The Topography of Reality: Sketching a Metapsychology of Secrets" (1971), in Abraham and Torok, *The Shell and the Kernel*, 157-61.

—, *The Shell and the Kernel: Renewals of Psychoanalysis*, trans. Nicholas T. Rand, Vol. I, Chicago: University of Chicago Press, 1994.

—, *The Wolf Man's Magic Word: A Cryptonomy* (1976), trans. Nicholas T. Rand, Minneapolis: University of Minnesota Press, 1986.

Acheson, James, and Sarah C.E. Ross, eds, *The Contemporary British Novel*, Edinburgh: Edinburgh University Press, 2005.

Adams, Timothy Dow, "'Bend Sinister': Duration in Elizabeth Bowen's *The House in Paris*", *International Fiction Review*, VII/1 (Winter 1980), 49-52.

Agamben, Giorgio, *Remnants of Auschwitz: The Witness and the Archive*, trans. Daniel Heller-Roazen, New York: Zone, 2002.

Aiken, Joan, "Demon Lovers", *Changing English*, IV/1 (1997), 67-79.

Alphen, Ernst van, *Caught by History: Holocaust Effects in Contemporary Art, Literature, and Theory*, Stanford, CA: Stanford University Press, 1998.

Alvarez, A., *Night: Night Life, Night Language, Sleep, and Dreams*, New York: W.W. Norton, 1995.

Ankersmit, Frank, *Sublime Historical Experience*, Stanford, CA: Stanford University Press, 2005.

Antze, Paul, and Michael Lambek, "Forecasting Memory", in Antze and Lambek, *Tense Past*, xi-xxxviii

—, eds, *Tense Past: Cultural Essays in Trauma and Memory*, New York: Routledge, 1996.

Apter, Terri, *Altered Loves: Mothers and Daughters During Adolescence*, Hertfordshire: Harvester Wheatsheaf, 1990.

Armstrong, Nancy, and Leonard Tennenhouse, eds, *The Violence of Representation: Literature and the History of Violence*, London: Routledge, 1989.

Ashford, David, "Children Asleep in the Underground: The Tube Shelters of Brandt and Moore", *Cambridge Quarterly*, XXXVI/4 (January 2007), 295-316.

Ashworth, Ann, "'But Why Was She Called Portia?': Judgment and Feeling in Bowen's *The Death of the Heart*", *Critique*, XXVIII (Spring 1987), 159-66.

Auerbach, Erich, *Mimesis: The Representation of Reality in Western Literature*, trans. Willard R. Trask, 50th anniversary edn, Princeton, NJ: Princeton University Press, 2003.

Austin, Allan E., *Elizabeth Bowen*, rev. edn, Boston: Twayne, 1989.

Bachelard, Gaston, *The Poetics of Space* (1958), trans. Maria Jolas, Boston, MA: Beacon, 1964.

Backus, Margaret Gayle, *The Gothic Family Romance: Heterosexuality, Child Sacrifice, and the Anglo-Irish Colonial Order*, Durham, NC: Duke University Press, 1999.

Balaev, Michelle, "Trends in Literary Trauma Theory", *Mosaic*, XLI/2 (June 2008), 149-66.

Barthes, Roland, *Camera Lucida: Reflections on Photography* (1981), trans. Richard Howard, London: Vintage, 2000.

—, *S/Z* (1973), trans. Richard Miller, Oxford: Blackwell, 1990.

Bates, Charlotte, "Hotel Histories: Modern Tourists, Modern Nomads and the Culture of Hotel-Consciousness", *Literature and History*, XII/2 (Autumn 2003), 62-75.

Bayley, John, *The Short Story: Henry James to Elizabeth Bowen*, Brighton: Harvester, 1988.

Beauman, Nicola, *A Very Great Profession: The Woman's Novel 1914-39*, London: Virago, 1983.

Beckett, J.C., *The Anglo-Irish Tradition*, London: Faber and Faber, 1976.

Begam, Richard, and Michael Valdez Moses, eds, *Modernism and Colonialism: British and Irish Literature, 1899-1939*, Durham, NC: Duke University Press, 2007.

Belau, Linda, and Petar Ramadanovic, eds, *Topologies of Trauma: Essays on the Limit of Knowledge and Memory*, New York: Other, 2002.

Bell, Amy, "Landscapes of Fear: Wartime London, 1939-1945", *Journal of British Studies*, XLVIII/1 (January 2009), 153-75.

Bellamy, Elizabeth J., *Affective Genealogies: Psychoanalysis, Postmodernism, and the "Jewish Question" after Auschwitz*, Lincoln, NE: University of Nebraska Press, 1997.

Bennett, Andrew, "Bowen and Modernism: The Early Novels", in Walshe, ed., *Elizabeth Bowen*, 27-39.

—, "Dendritic", *Oxford Literary Review*, XXIII (January 2002), 71-97.

—, ed., *Readers and Reading*, London: Longman, 1995.

Bennett, Andrew, and Nicholas Royle, "Torn-Off Senses", *Angelaki*, III/3 (June 1998), 153-58.

—, *Elizabeth Bowen and the Dissolution of the Novel: Still Lives*, London: Macmillan, 1995.

Berger, James, *After the End: Representations of Post-Apocalypse*, Minneapolis, MN: University of Minnesota Press, 1999.

Bergonzi, Bernard, *Wartime and Aftermath: English Literature and Its Background, 1939-60*, Oxford: Oxford University Press, 1993.

Berman, Jessica, "Ethical Folds: Ethics, Aesthetics, Woolf", *Modern Fiction Studies*, L/1 (Spring 2004), 151-72.

Bernard-Donals, Michael, "In Memoriam: Levinas, the Holocaust, and the Immemorial", *Mosaic*, XL/3 (September 2007), 1-16.

Bersani, Leo, *The Culture of Redemption*, Cambridge, MA: Harvard University Press, 1990.

—, *The Freudian Body: Psychoanalysis and Art*, New York: Columbia University Press, 1986.

Bettelheim, Bruno, *Freud and Man's Soul*, London: Hogarth, 1983.

—, *The Uses of Enchantment: The Meaning and Importance of Fairy Tales*, London: Penguin, 1976.

Bidney, Martin, "Nostalgic Narcissism in Comic and Tragic Perspectives: Elizabeth Bowen's Two Fictional Reworkings of a Tennyson Lyric", *Studies in Short Fiction*, XXXIII/1 (January 1996), 59-68.

Blodgett, Harriet, "The Necessary Child: *The House in Paris*", in Bloom, ed., *Elizabeth Bowen*, 63-79.

Bloom, Harold, "Introduction" in Bloom, ed., *Elizabeth Bowen*, 1-11.

—, ed., *Elizabeth Bowen*, New York: Chelsea House, 1987.

Boheemen-Saaf, Christine van, *Joyce, Derrida, Lacan, and the Trauma of History: Reading, Narrative and Postcolonialism*, Cambridge: Cambridge University Press, 1999.

Bollas, Christopher, *The Shadow of the Object: Psychoanalysis of the Unthought Known*, London: Free Association, 1987.

Botting, Fred, *Gothic*, London: Routledge, 1996.

Braidotti, Rosi, *Nomadic Subjects: Embodiment and Sexual Difference in Contemporary Feminist Theory*, New York: Columbia University Press, 1994.

Brannigan, John, *Orwell to the Present: Literature in England, 1945-2000*, Houndmills: Palgrave Macmillan, 2003.

Brassard, Geneviève, "Fast and Loose in Interwar London: Mobility and Sexuality in Elizabeth Bowen's *To the North*", *Women: A Cultural Review*, XVIII/3 (November 2007), 282-302.

Breen, Mary, "Autobiography as We Know It Now Is Artists' Work", in Walshe, ed., *Elizabeth Bowen*, 110-32.

Brewster, Scott, "Death and the Dinner Party: Hospitality and Hungry History in Joyce and Bowen", *Angelaki*, III/3 (June 1998), 59-68.

Briggs, Julia, "The Ghost Story", in Punter, ed., *A Companion to the Gothic*, 122-31.

—, "Resisting Nostalgia, Elizabeth Bowen's *A World of Love*", in Dowson, ed., *Women's Writing*, 29-37.

Brison, Susan J., "Trauma Narratives and the Remaking of the Self", in *Acts of Memory: Cultural Recall in the Present*, eds Mieke Bal, Jonathan V. Crewe, and Leo Spitzer, Hanover, NH: University Press of New England, 1999, 39-54.

Britzolakis, Christina, *Sylvia Plath and the Theatre of Mourning*, Oxford: Clarendon, 1999.

Brooke, Jocelyn, *Elizabeth Bowen*, London: Longmans, Green, 1952.

Brooke, Stephen, "War and the Nude: The Photography of Bill Brandt in the 1940s", *Journal of British Studies*, XLV (January 2006), 118-38.

Brooks, Peter, and Alex Woloch, eds, *Whose Freud?: The Place of Psychoanalysis in Contemporary Culture*, New Haven, CT: Yale University Press, 2000.

Brown, Spencer Curtis, "Foreword", in Bowen, *Pictures and Conversations*, vii-xlii.

Brown, Terence, *Ireland: A Social and Cultural History, 1922-2002*, 2nd edn, London: Harper Perennial, 2004.

Buccleugh, Stephen Hamilton, "The Dialogic of Narrative: The Use of Free Indirect Discourse in Elizabeth Bowen's 'The Return'", *South Central Review*, VII/2 (Summer 1990), 31-39.

Burgess, Anthony, "Treasures and Fetters", *Spectator*, 21 February 1964, 254.

Burrows, Victoria, *Whiteness and Trauma: The Mother-Daughter Knot in the Fiction of Jean Rhys, Jamaica Kincaid and Toni Morrison*, Houndmills: Palgrave Macmillan, 2004.

Buse, Peter, and Andrew Stott, "A Future for Haunting", in Buse and Stott, eds, *Ghosts*, 1-20.

—, eds, *Ghosts: Deconstruction, Psychoanalysis, History*, Houndmills: Macmillan, 1999.

Butler, Hubert, "Elizabeth Bowen: From *Escape from the Anthill*", in Walshe, ed., *Elizabeth Bowen Remembered*, 15-17.

Butler, Judith, "Giving an Account of Oneself", *Diacritics*, XXXI/4 (Winter 2001), 22-40.

—, *Precarious Life: The Powers of Mourning and Violence*, London: Verso, 2004.

Byatt, A.S., "Introduction", in Bowen, *The House in Paris*, 7-16.

Cahalan, James M., *The Irish Novel: A Critical History*, Dublin: Gill and Macmillan, 1988.

Calder, Robert L., "'A More Sinister Troth': Elizabeth Bowen's 'The

Demon Lover' as Allegory", *Studies in Short Fiction*, XXXI/1 (January 1994), 91-97.

Calinescu, Matei, *Rereading*, New Haven, CT: Yale University Press, 1993.

Campbell, Matthew, Jacqueline M. Labbe, and Sally Shuttleworth, eds, *Memory and Memorials: From the French Revolution to World War One*, New Brunswick: Transaction, 2004.

Caputo, John D., *The Prayers and Tears of Jacques Derrida: Religion Without Religion*, Bloomington, IN: Indiana University Press, 1997.

Carey, Maurice, "Places and People", in Walshe, ed., *Elizabeth Bowen Remembered*, 18-20.

Carroll, Joseph T., *Ireland in the War Years*, Newton Abbot: David and Charles, 1975.

Carroll, Lewis, *"Alice's Adventures in Wonderland" and "Through the Looking-Glass, and What Alice Found There"* (1865), ed. Roger Lancelyn Green, Oxford: Oxford University Press, 2008.

Caruth, Cathy, "Introduction", in Caruth, *Trauma*, 3-12.

—, "Parting Words: Trauma, Silence, and Survival", in Jacobs and Sussman, eds, *Acts of Narrative*, 47-61.

—, "Unclaimed Experience: Trauma and the Possibility of History", *Yale French Studies*, LXXIX (January 1991), 181-92.

—, *Unclaimed Experience: Trauma, Narrative, and History*, Baltimore, MD: Johns Hopkins University Press, 1996.

—, ed., *Trauma: Explorations in Memory*, Baltimore, MD: Johns Hopkins University Press, 1995.

Caserio, Robert L., "*The Heat of the Day*: Modernism and Narrative in Paul De Man and Elizabeth Bowen", *Modern Language Quarterly*, LIV/2 (June 1993), 263-84.

—, ed., *The Cambridge Companion to the Twentieth-Century English Novel*, Cambridge: Cambridge University Press, 2009.

Castricano, Jodey, *Cryptomimesis: The Gothic and Jacques Derrida's Ghost Writing*, Montreal: McGill-Queen's University Press, 2001.

Cavaliero, Glen, *The Supernatural and English Fiction*, Oxford: Oxford University Press, 1995.

Cavarero, Adriana, *Relating Narratives: Storytelling and Selfhood*, trans. Paul A. Kottman, London: Routledge, 1997.

Chamberlain, Mary, and Paul Thompson, eds, *Narrative and Genre*, London: Routledge, 1998.

Chambers, Ross, *Untimely Interventions: AIDS Writing, Testimonial, and the Rhetoric of Haunting*, Ann Arbor, MI: University of Michigan Press, 2004.

Chessman, Harriet S., "Women and Language in the Fiction of Elizabeth Bowen", *Twentieth Century Literature*, XXIX/1 (Spring 1983), 69-85.

Chodorow, Nancy, *The Reproduction of Mothering: Psychoanalysis and the Sociology of Gender*, Berkeley, CA: University of California Press, 1978.

Christensen, Lis, "A Reading of Elizabeth Bowen's 'A Day in the Dark'", *Irish University Review*, XXVII/2 (Autumn-Winter 1997), 299-309.

—, *Elizabeth Bowen: The Later Fiction*, Copenhagen: Museum Tusculanum, 2001.

Church, Margaret, "Social Consciousness in the Works of Elizabeth Bowen, Iris Murdoch and Mary Lavin", *College Literature*, VII/2 (Spring 1980), 158-63.

Cixous, Hélène, "Fiction and Its Phantoms: A Reading of Freud's *Das Unheimliche* (The 'Uncanny')", trans. Robert Dennomé, *New Literary History*, VII/3 (Spring 1976), 525-48, 619-45.

—, "Introduction to Lewis Carroll's *Through the Looking-Glass* and *The Hunting of the Snark*", trans. Marie Maclean, *New Literary History*, XIII/2 (Winter 1982), 231-51.

—, "Preface: On Stigmatexts", trans. Eric Prenowitz, in Cixous, *Stigmata*, xi-xvi.

—, "What is it O'Clock? Or the Door (We Never Enter)" (1994), trans. Catherine A.F. MacGillivray, in Cixous, *Stigmata*, 72-109.

—, "Without End, No, State of Drawingness, No, Rather: The Executioner's Taking Off" (1991), trans. Catherine A.F. MacGillivray, in Cixous, *Stigmata*, 25-40.

—, *Portrait of Jacques Derrida as a Young Jewish Saint*, trans. Beverley Bie Brahic, New York: Columbia University Press, 2004.

—, *Stigmata: Escaping Texts* (1998), London: Routledge, 2005.

—, *Three Steps on the Ladder of Writing*, trans. Sarah Cornell and Susan Sellers, New York: Columbia University Press, 1993.

Cixous, Hélène, and Jacques Derrida, *Veils*, trans. Geoffrey

Bennington, Stanford, CA: Stanford University Press, 2001.

Clej, Alina, *A Genealogy of the Modern Self: Thomas de Quincey and the Intoxication of Writing*, Stanford, CA: Stanford University Press, 1995.

Clewell, Tammy, "Consolation Refused: Virginia Woolf, the Great War, and Modernist Mourning", *Modern Fiction Studies*, L/1 (Spring 2004), 197-223.

—, "Mourning Beyond Melancholia: Freud's Psychoanalysis of Loss", *JAPA*, LII/1 (March 2004), 43-67.

Coates, John, "Elizabeth Bowen's *The Last September*: The Loss of the Past and the Modern Consciousness", *Durham University Journal*, LI (July 1990), 205-16.

—, "Emotional Need and Cultural Codes in *The House in Paris*", *Renascence*, XLVII/1 (Fall 1994), 11-29.

—, "The Misfortunes of Eva Trout", *Essays in Criticism*, XLVIII/1 (January 1998) 59-79.

—, "The Moral Argument of Elizabeth Bowen's Ghost Stories", *Renascence*, LII/4 (Summer 2000), 292-311.

—, *Social Discontinuity in the Novels of Elizabeth Bowen: The Conservative Quest*, New York: Edwin Mellen, 1998.

Coelsch-Foisner, Sabine, "Finding a Voice: Women Writing the Short Story (to 1945)", in Malcolm and Malcolm, eds, *A Companion to the British and Irish Short Story*, 96-113.

Cohen, Milton A., "Fatal Symbiosis: Modernism and the First World War", in Quinn and Trout, eds, *The Literature of the Great War Reconsidered*, 159-71.

Cohn, Dorrit, *Transparent Minds: Narrative Modes for Presenting Consciousness in Fiction*, Princeton, NJ: Princeton University Press, 1978.

Cole, Robert, *Propaganda, Censorship and Irish Neutrality in the Second World War*, Edinburgh: Edinburgh University Press, 2006.

Coles, Robert, *Irony in the Mind's Life: Essays on Novels by James Agee, Elizabeth Bowen, and George Eliot*, Charlottesville, VA: University Press of Virginia, 1974.

Concilio, Carmen, "Things That Do Speak in Elizabeth Bowen's *The Last September*", in *Moments of Moment: Aspects of the Literary Epiphany*, ed. Wim Tigges, Amsterdam: Rodopi, 1999, 279-92.

Connerton, Paul, *How Societies Remember*, Cambridge: Cambridge University Press, 1989.

Connolly, Claire, "(Be)longing: The Strange Place of Elizabeth Bowen's *Eva Trout*", in *Borderlands: Negotiating Boundaries in Post-Colonial Writing*, ed. Monika Reif-Hülser, Amsterdam: Rodopi, 1999, 135-43.

—, ed., *Theorizing Ireland*, New York: Palgrave Macmillan, 2003.

Cooke, Maeve, "The Ethics of Post-Holocaust Art: Reflections on Redemption and Representation", *German Life and Letters*, LIX/2 (April 2006), 266-79.

Corbin, Laurie, *The Mother Mirror: Self-Representation and the Mother-Daughter Relation in Colette, Simone De Beauvoir, and Marguerite Duras*, New York: Peter Lang, 1996.

Corcoran, Neil, "Discovery of a Lack: History and Ellipsis in Elizabeth Bowen's *The Last September*", *Irish University Review*, XXXI/2 (Autumn-Winter 2001), 315-33.

—, "Foreword", in Walshe, ed., *Elizabeth Bowen*, xi-xv.

—, "A Ghost of Style: The Aftermath of Anglo-Ireland in Elizabeth Bowen's *A World of Love*", *English*, LII (Summer 2003), 125-37.

—, *After Yeats and Joyce: Reading Modern Irish Literature*, Oxford: Oxford University Press, 1997.

—, *Elizabeth Bowen: The Enforced Return*, Oxford: Oxford University Press, 2004.

Corse, Edward, "British Propaganda in Neutral Eire after the Fall of France, 1940", *Contemporary British History*, XXII/2 (June 2008), 163-80.

Coughlan, Patricia, "'Not Like a Person at All': Bowen, the 1920s and 'The Dancing-Mistress'", in Walshe, ed., *Elizabeth Bowen*, 40-64.

—, "Women and Desire in the Work of Elizabeth Bowen", in Walshe, ed., *Sex, Nation and Dissent in Irish Writing*, 103-34.

Craig, Patricia, *Elizabeth Bowen*, Harmondsworth: Penguin, 1986.

Cronin, Gearoid, "The Big House and the Irish Landscape in the Work of Elizabeth Bowen", in Genet, ed., *The Big House in Ireland*, 143-61.

Cronin, John, *The Anglo-Irish Novel*, Vol. I, Belfast: Appletree, 1980.

Crowell, Ellen, "Ghosting the Llangollen Ladies: Female Intimacies, Ascendancy Exiles, and the Anglo-Irish Novel", *Eire-Ireland*, XXXIX/3-4 (Fall-Winter 2004), 202-27.

Culler, Jonathan, *The Literary in Theory*, Stanford, CA: Stanford University Press, 2007.

Cullingford, Elizabeth, "'Something Else': Gendering Onliness in Elizabeth Bowen's Early Fiction", *Modern Fiction Studies*, LIII/2 (Summer 2007), 276-305.

Currie, Mark, *About Time: Narrative, Fiction and the Philosophy of Time*, Edinburgh: Edinburgh University Press, 2007.

Daiches, David, "The Novels of Elizabeth Bowen", *English Journal*, XXXVIII/6 (June 1949), 305-13.

Dalsimer, Katherine, *Female Adolescence: Psychoanalytic Reflections on Literature*, New Haven, CT: Yale University Press, 1986.

Darwood, Nicola, *A World of Lost Innocence: The Fiction of Elizabeth Bowen*, Newcastle-upon-Tyne: Cambridge Scholars, 2012.

Davies, Alistair, and Alan Sinfield, eds, *British Culture of the Postwar: An Introduction to Literature and Society 1945-1999*, London: Routledge, 2000.

Davis, Colin, "*États Présents*: Hauntology, Spectres and Phantoms", *French Studies*, LIX/3 (July 2005), 373-79.

—, *After Poststructuralism: Reading, Stories and Theory*, London: Routledge, 2004.

—, *Haunted Subjects: Deconstruction, Psychoanalysis and the Return of the Dead*, Houndmills: Palgrave Macmillan, 2007.

Davis, Philip, *Memory and Writing: From Wordsworth to Lawrence*, Liverpool: Liverpool University Press, 1983.

Dawson, Graham, *Making Peace with the Past?: Memory, Trauma and the Irish Troubles*, Manchester: Manchester University Press, 2007.

Deane, Seamus, "Dumbness and Eloquence: A Note on English as We Write It in Ireland", in *Ireland and Postcolonial Theory*, eds Clare Carroll and Patricia King, Notre Dame, IN: University of Notre Dame Press, 2003, 109-21.

—, *Strange Country: Modernity and Nationhood in Irish Writing since 1790*, Oxford: Oxford University Press, 1997.

—, ed., *The Field Day Anthology of Irish Writing*, Vol. II, Derry: Field Day, 1991.

DeCoste, Damon Marcel, "The Literary Response to the Second World War", in Shaffer, ed., *A Companion to the British and Irish Novel*, 3-20.

Deer, Patrick, *Culture in Camouflage: War, Empire, and Modern British Literature*, Oxford: Oxford University Press, 2009.

Delaney, Paul, "'Acts of Remembrance': History, Anxiety and Elizabeth Bowen", *Études Irlandaises*, XXXI/1 (Spring 2006), 87-103.

Derrida, Jacques, "At This Very Moment in This Work Here I Am", trans. Ruben Berezdivin and Peggy Kamuf, in Derrida, *Psyche*, Vol. I, 143-90.

—, "... That Dangerous Supplement ..." (1967), trans. Gayatri Chakravorty Spivak, in Derrida, *Acts of Literature*, 76-109.

—, "*Ex Abrupto*", trans. Peggy Kamuf, in Derrida, *Psyche*, Vol. I, 262-63.

—, "Foreword", in Cixous, *Stigmata*, trans. Eric Prenowitz, ix-x.

—, "*Fors*: The Anglish Words of Nicolas Abraham and Maria Torok", trans. Barbara Johnson, in Abraham and Torok, eds, *The Wolf Man's Magic Word*, xi-xlviii.

—, "Freud and the Scene of Writing", trans. Jeffrey Mehlman, *Yale French Studies*, XLVIII (1972), 74-117.

—, "My Chances/*Mes Chances*: A Rendezvous with Some Epicurean Stereophonies", trans. Irene Harvey and Avital Ronell, in Derrida, *Psyche*, Vol. I, 344-76.

—, "'Le Parjure', *Perhaps*: Storytelling and Lying ('Abrupt Breaches of Syntax')", in Jacobs and Sussman, eds, *Acts of Narrative*, 195-234.

—, "*From* Shibboleth: For Paul Celan" (1984), trans. Joshua Wilner, in Derrida, *Acts of Literature*, 370-413.

—, "Telepathy", trans. Nicholas Royle, *Oxford Literary Review*, X/1-2 (1988), 3-41.

—, *Acts of Literature*, ed. Derek Attridge, New York: Routledge, 1992.

—, *Archive Fever: A Freudian Impression*, trans. Eric Prenowitz, Chicago: University of Chicago Press, 1995.

—, *A Derrida Reader: Between the Blinds*, ed. Peggy Kamuf, New York: Columbia University Press, 1991.

—, *The Gift of Death*, trans. David Wills, Chicago: University of Chicago Press, 1995.

—, *Jacques Derrida*, trans. Geoffrey Bennington, Chicago: University of Chicago Press, 1993.

—, *Mémoires for Paul de Man*, trans. Cecile Lindsay, Jonathan Culler, Eduardo Cadava and Peggy Kamuf, rev. edn, New York: Columbia University Press, 1989.

—, *Of Grammatology* (1967), trans. Gayatri Chakravorty Spivak, corr. edn, Baltimore, MD: Johns Hopkins University Press, 1997.

—, *Paper Machine*, trans. Rachel Bowlby, Stanford, CA: Stanford University Press, 2005.

—, *The Politics of Friendship* (1994), trans. George Collins, London: Verso, 2005.

—, *The Post Card: From Socrates to Freud and Beyond*, trans. Alan Bass, Chicago: University of Chicago Press, 1987.

—, *Psyche: Inventions of the Other*, eds Peggy Kamuf and Elizabeth Rottenberg, Vol. I (1987), Stanford, CA: Stanford University Press, 2007.

—, *Psyche: Inventions of the Other*, eds Peggy Kamuf and Elizabeth Rottenberg, Vol. II (1987), Stanford, CA: Stanford University Press, 2008.

—, *Spectres of Marx: The State of the Debt, the Work of Mourning, and the New International*, trans. Peggy Kamuf, New York: Routledge, 1994.

—, *Writing and Difference* (1967), trans. Alan Bass, London: Routledge, 2001.

Derrida, Jacques, and Maurizio Ferraris, *A Taste for the Secret*, eds Giacomo Donis and David Webb, trans. Giacomo Donis, Cambridge: Polity, 2001.

DiBasio, Becky, "The British and Irish Ghost Story and Tale of the Supernatural: 1880-1945", in Malcolm and Malcolm, eds, *A Companion to the British and Irish Short Story*, 81-95.

DiBattista, Maria, "Elizabeth Bowen and the Maternal Sublime", in *Troubled Legacies: Narrative and Inheritance*, ed. Allan Hepburn, Toronto: University of Toronto Press, 2007, 219-38.

—, "Elizabeth Bowen's Troubled Modernism", in Begam and Moses, eds, *Modernism and Colonialism*, 226-45.

Dillon, Sarah, "Elizabeth Bowen: 'The Demon Lover' and

'Mysterious Kôr'", in Malcolm and Malcolm, eds, *A Companion to the British and Irish Short Story*, 236-43.

Doody, Noreen, "Elizabeth Bowen: A Short Biography", in Walshe, ed., *Elizabeth Bowen*, 1-11.

Dorenkamp, Angela G., "'Fall or Leap': Bowen's *The Heat of the Day*", *Critique*, X/3 (1968), 13-21.

Douglass, Ana, and Thomas A. Vogler, eds, *Witness and Memory: The Discourse of Trauma*, New York: Routledge, 2003.

Dowson, Jane, ed., *Women's Writing, 1945-60: After the Deluge*, Houndmills: Palgrave Macmillan, 2003.

Dowson, Jane, and Steven Earnshaw, eds, *Postmodern Subjects/Postmodern Texts*, Amsterdam: Rodopi, 1995.

Draaisma, Douwe, *Metaphors of Memory: A History of Ideas About the Mind*, trans. Paul Vincent, Cambridge: Cambridge University Press, 2000.

Duggan, John P., *Neutral Ireland and the Third Reich*, Dublin: Gill and Macmillan, 1985.

Dukes, Thomas, "Desire Satisfied: War and Love in *The Heat of the Day* and *Moon Tiger*", *War, Literature, and the Arts*, III/1 (Spring 1991), 75-97.

Dunleavy, Janet Egleson, "The Subtle Satire of Elizabeth Bowen and Mary Lavin", *Tulsa Studies in Women's Literature*, II/1 (Spring 1983), 69-82.

Eagleton, Terry, "Changing the Question", in Connolly, ed., *Theorizing Ireland*, 76-90.

—, *Heathcliff and the Great Hunger: Studies in Irish Literature*, London: Verso, 1995.

—, *Sweet Violence: The Idea of the Tragic*, Malden, MA: Blackwell, 2003.

Eberwein, Robert T., *Film and the Dream Screen: A Sleep and a Forgetting*, Princeton, NJ: Princeton University Press, 1984.

Edkins, Jenny, *Trauma and the Memory of Politics*, Cambridge: Cambridge University Press, 2003.

Ellmann, Maud, "Bad Timing", in Freud, *On Murder, Mourning and Melancholia*, vii-xxvii.

—, "Elizabeth Bowen: The Shadowy Fifth", in Mengham and Reeve, eds, *The Fiction of the 1940s: Stories of Survival*, 1-25.

—, *Elizabeth Bowen: The Shadow Across the Page*, Edinburgh: Edinburgh University Press, 2003.

—, ed., *Psychoanalytic Literary Criticism*, London: Longman, 1994.

Eng, David L., and David Kazanjian, eds, *Loss: The Politics of Mourning*, Berkeley, CA: University of California Press, 2003.

English, James F., ed., *A Concise Companion to Contemporary British Fiction*, Oxford: Blackwell, 2006.

Esty, Jed, "Virgins of Empire: *The Last September* and the Antidevelopmental Plot", *Modern Fiction Studies*, LIII/2 (Summer 2007), 257-75.

Ettinger, Bracha Lichtenberg, "Wit(h)nessing Trauma and the Matrixial Gaze: From Phantasm to Trauma, from Phallic Structure to Matrixial Sphere", *Parallax*, VII/4 (2001), 89-114.

—, *The Matrixial Borderspace*, ed. Brian Massumi, Minneapolis: University of Minnesota Press, 2006.

Feigel, Lara, *The Love-Charm of Bombs: Restless Lives in the Second World War*, London: Bloomsbury, 2013.

Felman, Shoshana, "To Open the Question", *Yale French Studies*, LV/LVI (1977), 5-10.

—, "Turning the Screw of Interpretation", *Yale French Studies*, LV/LVI (1977), 94-207.

Felman, Shoshana, and Dori Laub, *Testimony: Crises of Witnessing in Literature, Psychoanalysis, and History*, New York: Routledge, 1992.

Fisk, Robert, *In Time of War: Ireland, Ulster and the Price of Neutrality, 1939-45*, London: Andre Deutsch, 1983.

Flax, Jane, *Thinking Fragments: Psychoanalysis, Feminism, and Postmodernism in the Contemporary West*, Berkeley, CA: University of California Press, 1990.

Fletcher, John, and Andrew Benjamin, eds, *Abjection, Melancholia, and Love: The Work of Julia Kristeva*, London: Routledge, 1990.

Fogarty, Anne, "'The Horror of the Unlived Life': Mother-Daughter Relationships in Contemporary Irish Women's Fiction", in Giorgio, ed., *Writing Mothers and Daughters*, 85-118.

—, "Ireland and English Fiction", in Caserio, ed., *The Cambridge Companion to the Twentieth-Century English Novel*, 102-13.

Fogu, Claudio, and Wulf Kansteiner, "The Politics of Memory and the Poetics of History", in *The Politics of Memory in Postwar Europe*, eds Richard Ned Lebow, Wulf Kansteiner and Claudio Fogu, Durham, NC: Duke University Press, 2006, 284-310 .

Foster, R. F., "Irish and Regional: Locale in Elizabeth Bowen's Writing", in Walshe, ed., *Elizabeth Bowen Remembered*, 21-27.

—, *The Irish Story: Telling Tales and Making It Up in Ireland*, London: Penguin, 2001.

—, *Modern Ireland: 1600-1972*, London: Allen Lane, 1988.

—, *Paddy and Mr Punch: Connections in Irish and English History*, London: Penguin, 1993.

Foucault, Michel, *Language, Counter-Memory, Practice: Selected Essays and Interviews*, trans. Donald F. Bouchard and Sherry Simon, ed. Donald F. Bouchard, Oxford: Basil Blackwell, 1977.

Franks, Jill, "Sex, Guns, and Death: Deborah Warner's Adaptation of *The Last September*", *New Hibernia Review*, X/3 (Autumn 2006), 122-36.

Fraustino, Daniel V., "Elizabeth Bowen's 'The Demon Lover': Psychosis or Seduction?", *Studies in Short Fiction*, XVII/4 (Fall 1980), 483-87.

Freedman, Ariela, *Death, Men, and Modernism: Trauma and Narrative in British Fiction from Hardy to Woolf*, New York: Routledge, 2003.

Freud, Sigmund, "Beyond the Pleasure Principle" (1920), in Freud, *The Essentials of Psycho-Analysis*, 218-68.

—, "Family Romances" (1909), in Freud, *The Uncanny*, 35-41.

—, "Inhibitions, Symptoms and Anxiety" (1926), in *The Standard Edition of the Complete Psychological Works of Sigmund Freud*, trans. and eds James Strachey and Anna Freud, Vol. XX, London: Hogarth, 1953-73.

—, "Moses and Monotheism, An Outline of Psychoanalysis and Other Works", in *The Standard Edition of the Complete Psychological Works of Sigmund Freud*, trans. and eds James Strachey and Anna Freud, Vol. XXIII (1937-1939), London: Vintage, 2001.

—, "Mourning and Melancholia" (1917), in Freud, *On Murder, Mourning and Melancholia*, 203-18.

—, "On Dreams" (1901), in Freud, *The Essentials of Psycho-Analysis*, 81-125.

—, "Repression" (1915), in Freud, *The Essentials of Psycho-Analysis*, 523-33.

—, "Timely Reflections on War and Death" (1915), in Freud, *On Murder, Mourning and Melancholia*, 169-94.
—, "The Uncanny" (1919), in Freud, *The Uncanny*, 121-62.
—, *The Essentials of Psycho-Analysis*, trans. James Strachey, ed. Anna Freud, London: Vintage, 2005.
—, *General Psychological Theory* (1925), New York: Touchstone, 1997.
—, *The Interpretation of Dreams* (1899), trans. Joyce Crick, Oxford: Oxford University Press, 1999.
—, *On Murder, Mourning and Melancholia*, trans. Shaun Whiteside, London: Penguin, 2005.
—, *The Uncanny*, trans. David McLintock, London: Penguin, 2003.
Friedlander, Saul, ed., *Probing the Limits of Representation: Nazism and the "Final Solution"*, Cambridge, MA: Harvard University Press, 1992.
Gallop, Jane, *Feminism and Psychoanalysis: The Daughter's Seduction*, London: Macmillan, 1982.
Gana, Nouri, "Revolutionaries Without a Revolution: The Case of Julia Kristeva", *College Literature*, XXXI/4 (Fall 2004), 188-202.
Garber, Majorie B., *Dream in Shakespeare: From Metaphor to Metamorphosis*, New Haven, CT: Yale University Press, 1974.
Gavin, Adrienne, "Living in a World of Make-Believe: Fantasy, Female Identity, and Modern Short Stories by Women in the British Tradition", in *Postmodern Approaches to the Short Story*, eds Farhat Iftekharrudin, Joseph Boyden, Joseph Longo and Mary Rohrberger, Westport, CT: Greenwood, 2003, 121-32.
Genet, Jacqueline, ed., *The Big House in Ireland: Reality and Representation*, Kerry: Brandon, 1991.
Ghost Dance, dir. Ken McMullen, Other Cinema, 1983.
Gill, Richard, "The Country House in a Time of Troubles", in Bloom, ed., *Elizabeth Bowen*, 51-61.
Gilmore, Leigh, *The Limits of Autobiography: Trauma and Testimony*, Ithaca, NY: Cornell University Press, 2001.
Giobbi, Giuliana, "A Blurred Picture: Adolescent Girls Growing Up in Fanny Burney, George Eliot, Rosamond Lehmann, Elizabeth Bowen and Dacia Maraini", *Journal of European Studies*, XXV/2 (June 1995), 141-64.
Giorgio, Adalgisa, "Writing the Mother-Daughter Relationship:

Psychoanalysis, Culture, and Literary Criticism", in Giorgio, ed., *Writing Mothers and Daughters*, 11-45.

—, ed., *Writing Mothers and Daughters: Renegotiating the Mother in Western European Narratives by Women*, New York: Berghahn, 2002.

Glendinning, Victoria, "Gardens and Gardening in the Writings of Elizabeth Bowen", in Walshe, ed., *Elizabeth Bowen Remembered*, 28-34.

—, *Elizabeth Bowen: Portrait of a Writer* (1977), Harmondsworth: Penguin, 1985.

Glendinning, Victoria, with Judith Robertson, eds, *Love's Civil War: Elizabeth Bowen and Charles Ritchie, Letters and Diaries, 1941-1973*, London: Simon and Schuster, 2008.

Glover, David, and Cora Kaplan, *Genders*, London: Routledge, 2000.

Gonzalez, Alexander G., "Elizabeth Bowen's 'Her Table Spread': A Joycean Irish Story", *Studies in Short Fiction*, XXX/3 (Summer 1993), 343-48.

Graham, Colin, *Deconstructing Ireland: Identity, Theory, Culture*, Edinburgh: Edinburgh University Press, 2001.

Gray, Peter, and Kendrick Oliver, "Introduction", in Gray and Oliver, eds, *The Memory of Catastrophe*, 1-18.

—, eds, *The Memory of Catastrophe*, Manchester: Manchester University Press, 2004.

Greaves, Richard, "Responses to War: 1914-18 and 1939-45", in Malcolm and Malcolm, eds, *A Companion to the British and Irish Short Story*, 35-50.

Greene, Gayle, "Feminist Fiction and the Uses of Memory", *Signs*, XVI/2 (Winter 1991), 290-321.

Greene, George, "Elizabeth Bowen: The Sleuth Who Bugged Tea Cups", *Virginia Quarterly Review*, LXVII/4 (Autumn 1991), 604-18.

Grosz, Elizabeth, *Jacques Lacan: A Feminist Introduction*, London: Routledge, 1990.

—, *Sexual Subversions: Three French Feminists*, Sydney: Allen and Unwin, 1989.

Grubgeld, Elizabeth, "Cultural Autobiography and the Female Subject: The Genre of the Patrilineal History and the Lifewriting of Elizabeth Bowen", *Genre*, XXVII/3 (Fall 1994), 209-26.

Gunn, Daniel, *Psychoanalysis and Fiction: An Exploration of Literary and Psychoanalytic Borders*, Cambridge: Cambridge University Press, 1988.

Hand, Derek, "Ghosts from Our Future: Bowen and the Unfinished Business of Living", in Walshe, ed., *Elizabeth Bowen*, 65-76.

Hanson, Clare, "The Free Story", in Bloom, ed., *Elizabeth Bowen*, 139-51.

—, "Little Girls and Large Women: Representations of the Female Body in Elizabeth Bowen's Later Fiction", in *Body Matters: Feminism, Textuality, Corporeality*, eds Avril Horner, and Angela Keane, Manchester: Manchester University Press, 2000, 185-98.

—, *A Cultural History of Pregnancy: Pregnancy, Medicine and Culture, 1750-2000*, Houndmills: Palgrave Macmillan, 2004.

—, *Hysterical Fictions: The "Woman's Novel" in the Twentieth Century*, Houndmills: Macmillan, 2000.

Hapgood, Lynne, and Nancy L. Paxton, eds, *Outside Modernism: In Pursuit of the English Novel, 1900-30*, Houndmills: Macmillan, 2000.

Harkness, Bruce, "The Fiction of Elizabeth Bowen", *English Journal*, XLIV/9 (December 1955), 499-506.

Hartman, Geoffrey, *The Longest Shadow: In the Aftermath of the Holocaust*, Bloomington, IN: Indiana University Press, 1996.

—, *Scars of the Spirit: The Struggle Against Inauthenticity*, New York: Palgrave Macmillan, 2002.

Haughton, Hugh, "Introduction", in Bowen, *To the North*, vii-xix.

—, "Introduction", in Freud, *The Uncanny*, vii-lx.

Head, Dominic, *The Cambridge Introduction to Modern British Fiction, 1950-2000*, Cambridge: Cambridge University Press, 2002.

The Heat of the Day, dir. Christopher Morahan, WGBH Educational Foundation, 1991.

Heath, William, "The Jacobean Melodrama of *To the North*", in Bloom, ed., *Elizabeth Bowen*, 27-38.

—, *Elizabeth Bowen: An Introduction to Her Novels*, Madison: University of Wisconsin Press, 1961.

Henke, Suzette A., *Shattered Subjects: Trauma and Testimony in Women's Life-Writing*, London: Macmillan, 2000.

Hepburn, Allan, *Intrigue: Espionage and Culture*, New Haven, CT: Yale University Press, 2005.

Herman, Nini, *Too Long a Child: The Mother-Daughter Dyad*, London: Free Association, 1989.

Herr, Cheryl, "The Erotics of Irishness", *Critical Quarterly*, XVII/1 (Autumn 1990), 1-34.

Hirsch, Marianne, "The Generation of Postmemory", *Poetics Today*, XXIX/1 (Spring 2008), 103-28.

—, *Family Frames: Photography, Narrative, and Postmemory*, Cambridge, MA: Harvard University Press, 1997.

—, *The Mother/Daughter Plot: Narrative, Psychoanalysis, Feminism*, Bloomington: Indiana University Press, 1989.

Holland, Nancy J., "The Death of the Other/Father: A Feminist Reading of Derrida's Hauntology", *Hypatia*, XVI/1 (Winter 2001), 64-71.

Hoogland, Renée C., "Elizabeth Bowen: Unconscious Undertows: Queer Perspectives on *Friends and Relations*", in Quinn, ed., *Recharting the Thirties*, 82-101.

—, *Elizabeth Bowen: A Reputation in Writing*, New York: New York University Press, 1994.

Hooper, Brad, "Elizabeth Bowen's 'The Happy Autumn Fields': A Dream or Not?", *Studies in Short Fiction*, XXI/2 (Spring 1984), 151-53.

Hopkins, Chris, "Elizabeth Bowen", *Review of Contemporary Fiction*, XXI/2 (Summer 2001), 114-49.

—, "Elizabeth Bowen: Realism, Modernism and Gendered Identity in Her Novels of the 1930s", *Journal of Gender Studies*, IV/3 (1995), 271-79.

—, *English Fiction in the 1930s: Language, Genre, History*, London: Continuum, 2006.

Horvitz, Deborah M., *Literary Trauma: Sadism, Memory, and Sexual Violence in American Women's Fiction*, Albany, NY: State University of New York Press, 2000.

Howlett, Jana, and Rod Mengham, eds, *The Violent Muse: Violence and the Artistic Imagination in Europe, 1910-1939*, Manchester: Manchester University Press, 1994.

Humble, Nicola, *The Feminine Middlebrow Novel, 1920s-1950s: Class, Domesticity, and Bohemianism*, Oxford: Oxford University Press, 2004.

Huyssen, Andreas, *Present Pasts: Urban Palimpsests and the Politics of Memory*, Stanford, CA: Stanford University Press, 2003.

Ingelbien, Raphael, "A Girl in the Forties: Larkin and the Politics of World War Two", *Critical Survey*, XIII/1 (January 2001), 80-93.

—, "Gothic Genealogies: *Dracula*, *Bowen's Court*, and Anglo-Irish Psychology", *ELH*, LII/4 (Winter 2003), 1089-105.

Inglesby, Elizabeth C., "'Expressive Objects': Elizabeth Bowen's Narrative Materializes", *Modern Fiction Studies*, LIII/2 (Summer 2007), 306-33.

Ingman, Heather, *Twentieth-Century Fiction by Irish Women: Nation and Gender*, Aldershot: Ashgate, 2007.

—, *Women's Fiction Between the Wars: Mothers, Daughters and Writing*, New York: St Martin's, 1998.

Ingram, Forrest L., *Representative Short Story Cycles of the Twentieth Century*, The Hague: Mouton, 1971.

Innes, C.L., "Custom, Ceremony and Innocence: Elizabeth Bowen's *The Last September*", in *Troubled Histories, Troubled Fictions: Twentieth-Century Anglo-Irish Prose*, eds Theo D'haen and José Lanters, Amsterdam: Rodopi, 1995), 105-18.

Irigaray, Luce, *The Irigaray Reader*, ed. Margaret Whitford, Oxford: Basil Blackwell, 1991.

—, *Key Writings*, London: Continuum, 2004.

Irwin-Zarecka, Iwona, *Frames of Remembrance: The Dynamics of Collective Memory*, New Brunswick, NJ: Transaction, 1994.

Jacobs, Carol, and Henry Sussman, eds, *Acts of Narrative*, Stanford, CA: Stanford University Press, 2003.

Jacobus, Mary, *First Things: The Maternal Imaginary in Literature, Art, and Psychoanalysis*, New York: Routledge, 1995.

—, *Psychoanalysis and the Scene of Reading*, Oxford: Oxford University Press, 1999.

James, David, "The New Purism", *Textual Practice*, XXI/4 (2007), 687-714.

Jeffares, A. Norman, *Anglo-Irish Literature*, Dublin: Gill and Macmillan, 1982.

Joannou, Maroula, *Ladies, Please Don't Smash These Windows:*

Women's Writing, Feminist Consciousness, and Social Change, 1918-38, Providence, RI: Berg, 1995.

—, ed., *Women Writers of the 1930s: Gender, Politics and History*, Edinburgh: Edinburgh University Press, 1999.

Johnson, Barbara, "Translator's Note", in Abraham and Torok, eds, *The Wolf Man's Magic Word*, xi-xlviii.

—, *Mother Tongues: Sexuality, Trials, Motherhood, Translation*, Cambridge, MA: Harvard University Press, 2003.

Johnson, Toni O'Brien, "Light and Enlightenment in Elizabeth Bowen's Irish Novels", *ARIEL*, XVIII/2 (April 1987), 47-62.

Jones, Ernest, *On the Nightmare*, 2nd edn (1931), New York: Liveright, 1951.

Jones, Hester, "Triumphant Obstination: Reading Adrienne Rich and Elizabeth Bowen", in *Real Voices on Reading*, ed. Philip Davis, Houndmills: Macmillan, 1997, 103-21.

Jordan, Heather Bryant, "A Bequest of Her Own: The Reinvention of Elizabeth Bowen", *New Hibernia Review*, XII/2 (Summer 2008), 46-62.

—, *How Will the Heart Endure: Elizabeth Bowen and the Landscape of War*, Ann Arbor: University of Michigan Press, 1992.

Jouve, Nicole Ward, *Female Genesis: Creativity, Self and Gender*, Cambridge: Polity, 1998.

Jung, C.G., *Dreams*, trans. R.F.C. Hull, London: Ark, 1982.

Kaplan, E. Ann, *Trauma Culture: The Politics of Terror and Loss in Media and Literature*, New Brunswick, NJ: Rutgers University Press, 2005.

Kelly, Gary, "Gender and Memory in Post-Revolutionary Women's Writing", in Campbell *et al.*, eds, *Memory and Memorials*, 119-31.

Kelly, Marian, "The Power of the Past: Structural Nostalgia in Elizabeth Bowen's *The House in Paris* and *The Little Girls*", *Style*, XXXVI/1 (Spring 2002), 1-18.

Kemp, Sandra, "'But How Describe a World Seen Without a Self?': Feminism, Fiction and Modernism", *Critical Quarterly*, XXXII/1 (March 1990), 99-118.

Kenney, Edwin J., *Elizabeth Bowen*, London: Associated University Press, 1975.

Kiberd, Declan, *Inventing Ireland: The Literature of the Modern Nation*, London: Vintage, 1996.

—, *The Irish Writer and the World*, Cambridge: Cambridge University Press, 2005.

Killeen, Jarlath, "Irish Gothic: A Theoretical Introduction", *Irish Journal of Gothic and Horror Studies*, 1 (2006), <http://irishgothichorrorjournal.homestead.com/jarlath.html>.

King, Nicola, *Memory, Narrative, Identity: Remembering the Self*, Edinburgh: Edinburgh University Press, 2000.

Kitagawa, Yoriko, "Anticipating the Postmodern Self: Elizabeth Bowen's *The Death of the Heart*", *English Studies*, LXXXI/5 (2000), 484-96.

Klein, Melanie, *Contributions to Psycho-Analysis: 1921-1945*, London: Hogarth, 1948.

—, *Envy and Gratitude: A Study of Unconscious Sources*, London: Tavistock, 1957.

Knaap, Ewout van der, ed., *Uncovering the Holocaust: The International Reception of "Night and Fog"*, London: Wallflower, 2006.

Krapp, Peter, *Deja Vu: Aberrations of Cultural Memory*, Minneapolis: University of Minnesota Press, 2004.

Kreilkamp, Vera, "Bowen: Ascendancy Modernist", in Walshe, ed., *Elizabeth Bowen*, 12-26.

Krell, David Farrell, *The Purest of Bastards: Works of Mourning, Art, and Affirmation in the Thought of Jacques Derrida*, University Park: Pennsylvania State University Press, 2000.

Kremer, S. Lillian, *Women's Holocaust Writing: Memory and Imagination*, Lincoln: University of Nebraska Press, 2001.

Kristeva, Julia, "Stabat Mater" (1983), trans. Leon S. Roudiez, in *Kristeva Reader*, 160-86.

—, "Women's Time", trans. Alice Jardine and Harry Blake, *Signs*, VII/1 (Autumn 1981), 13-35.

—, *Black Sun: Depression and Melancholia*, trans. Leon S. Roudiez, New York: Columbia University Press, 1989.

—, *The Kristeva Reader*, ed. Toril Moi, Oxford: Basil Blackwell, 1986.

—, *Powers of Horror: An Essay on Abjection*, trans. Leon S. Roudiez, New York: Columbia University Press, 1982.

—, *Strangers to Ourselves*, trans. Leon S. Roudiez, Hemel Hempstead: Harvester Wheatsheaf, 1991.

Lacan, Jacques, "Seminar on 'The Purloined Letter'", trans. Jeffrey Mehlman, *Yale French Studies*, XLVIII (1972), 39-72.

—, *Écrits: A Selection*, trans. Alan Sheridan (1966), London: Routledge, 2001.

Lacan, Jacques, Jacques-Alain Miller, and James Hulbert, "Desire and the Interpretation of Desire in *Hamlet*", *Yale French Studies*, LV/LVI (1977), 11-52.

LaCapra, Dominick, *History and Memory after Auschwitz*, Ithaca, NY: Cornell University Press, 1998.

—, *History in Transit: Experience, Identity, Critical Theory*, Ithaca, NY: Cornell University Press, 2004.

—, *Writing History, Writing Trauma*, Baltimore, MD: Johns Hopkins University Press, 2001.

Laigle, Deirdre M., "Images of the Big House in Elizabeth Bowen: *The Last September*", *Cahiers du Centre d'Etudes Irlandaises*, IX (1984), 61-80.

Laing, Kathryn, "Virginia Woolf in Ireland: A Short Voyage Out", *South Carolina Review*, XXXIV/1 (Fall 2001), 180-87.

Lang, Berel, ed., *Writing and the Holocaust*, New York: Holmes and Meier, 1988.

Lassner, Phyllis, "'The Past Is a Burning Pattern': Elizabeth Bowen's *The Last September*", *Eire-Ireland*, XXI/1 (Spring 1986), 40-54.

—, "Reimagining the Arts of War: Language and History in Elizabeth Bowen's *The Heat of the Day* and Rose Macaulay's *The World My Wilderness*", *Perspectives on Contemporary Literature*, XIV (1988), 30-38.

—, *Elizabeth Bowen*, London: Macmillan, 1990.

—, *Elizabeth Bowen: A Study of the Short Fiction*, New York: Twayne, 1991.

The Last September, dir. Deborah Warner, Trimark, 1999.

Lawson, Tom, "'The Free-Masonry of Sorrow'? English National Identities and the Memorialization of the Great War in Britain, 1919-1931", *History and Memory*, XX/1 (Spring/Summer 2008), 89-120.

Leavey, Jr., John P., "*Destinerrance*: The Apotropocalyptics of Translation", in *Deconstruction and Philosophy: The Texts of Jacques Derrida*, ed. John Sallis, Chicago: University of Chicago Press, 1987, 33-43.

Lee, Hermione, "The Placing of Loss: Elizabeth Bowen's *To the North*", *Essays in Criticism*, XXVIII (April 1978), 129-42.

—, *Body Parts: Essays in Life-Writing*, London: Chatto and Windus, 2005.

—, *Elizabeth Bowen*, rev. edn, London: Vintage, 1999.

Leerssen, Joep, "Monument and Trauma: Varieties of Remembrance", in McBride, ed., *History and Memory in Modern Ireland*, 204-22.

—, *Remembrance and Imagination: Patterns in the Historical and Literary Representation of Ireland in the Nineteenth Century*, Cork: Cork University Press, 1996.

Lennon, Mary, Marie McAdam, and Joanna O'Brien, *Across the Water: Irish Women's Lives in Britain*, London: Virago, 1988.

Leray, Josette, "Elizabeth Bowen's *A World of Love*", in Genet, eds, *The Big House in Ireland*, 163-78.

Leys, Ruth, "Image and Trauma", *Science in Context*, XIX/1 (March 2006), 137-49.

—, *Trauma: A Genealogy*, Chicago: University of Chicago Press, 2000.

Lifton, Robert Jay, *The Broken Connection: On Death and the Continuity of Life*, Washington, DC: American Psychiatric Press, 1979.

Light, Alison, *Forever England: Femininity, Literature and Conservatism Between the Wars*, London: Routledge, 1991.

Lippmann, Paul, "The Canary in the Mind: On the Fate of Dreams in Psychoanalysis and in Contemporary Culture", *American Journal of Psychoanalysis*, LXVI/2 (June 2006), 113-30.

Liu, Alan, "The New Historicism and the Work of Mourning", in *The Wordsworthian Enlightenment: Romantic Poetry and the Ecology of Reading*, eds Helen Regueiro Elam and Frances Ferguson, Baltimore, MD: Johns Hopkins University Press, 2005, 149-57.

Lomas, David, *The Haunted Self: Surrealism, Psychoanalysis, Subjectivity*, New Haven, CT: Yale University Press, 2000.

Lonergan, Patrick, "Irish Short Fiction: 1880-1945", in Malcolm and Malcolm, eds, *A Companion to the British and Irish Short Story*, 51-64.

Loraux, Nicole, *Mothers in Mourning, with the essay "Of Amnesty and Its Opposite"*, trans. Corinne Pache, Ithaca, NY: Cornell University Press, 1998.

Lounsberry, Barbara, Susan Lohafer, Mary Rohrberger, Stephen Pett, and R.C. Feddersen, eds, *The Tales We Tell: Perspectives on the Short Story*, Westport, CT: Greenwood, 1998.

Lubbers, Klaus, "Continuity and Change in Irish Fiction: The Case of the Big-House Novel", in Rauchbauer, ed., *Ancestral Voices*, 17-29.

Luckhurst, Roger, *The Trauma Question*, London: Routledge, 2008.

Lyons, F.S.L., *Culture and Anarchy in Ireland, 1890-1939*, Oxford: Clarendon, 1979.

McBride, Ian, ed., *History and Memory in Modern Ireland*, Cambridge: Cambridge University Press, 2001.

MacCannell, Juliet Flower, *Figuring Lacan: Criticism and the Cultural Unconscious*, London: Croom Helm, 1986.

MacCarthy, Robert, "Bowen Religion", in Walshe, ed., *Elizabeth Bowen Remembered*, 35-39.

McConville, Michael, *Ascendancy to Oblivion: The Story of the Anglo-Irish*, London: Quartet, 1986.

McCormack, W.J., "Irish Gothic and After (1820-1945)", in Deane, ed., *The Field Day Anthology of Irish Writing*, 831-949.

—, *Dissolute Characters: Irish Literary History Through Balzac, Sheridan Le Fanu, Yeats and Bowen*, Manchester: Manchester University Press, 1993.

MacCurdy, Marian Mesrobian, *The Mind's Eye: Image and Memory in Writing About Trauma*, Amherst: University of Massachussetts Press, 2007.

MacDonald, Ronald R., ed., *The Burial Places of Memory: Epic Underworlds in Virgil, Dante, and Milton*, Amherst: University of Massachusetts Press, 1987.

McDowell, Alfred, "*The Death of the Heart* and the Human Dilemma", *Modern Language Studies*, VIII/2 (Spring 1978), 5-16.

McGowan, Martha, "The Enclosed Garden in Elizabeth Bowen's *A World of Love*", *Eire-Ireland*, XVI/1 (Spring 1981), 55-70.

McHugh, Roger, and Maurice Harmon, *Short History of Anglo-Irish Literature: From Its Origins to the Present Day*, Dublin: Wolfhound, 1982.

MacKay, Marina, "World War II, the Welfare State, and Postwar 'Humanism'", in Caserio, ed., *The Cambridge Companion to the Twentieth-Century English Novel*, 146-62.

—, ed., *The Cambridge Companion to the Literature of World War II*, Cambridge: Cambridge University Press, 2009.

MacKay, Marina, and Lyndsey Stonebridge, eds, *British Fiction after Modernism: The Novel at Mid-Century*, Houndmills: Palgrave Macmillan, 2007.

McMahon, Paul, *British Spies and Irish Rebels: British Intelligence and Ireland, 1916-1945*, Woodbridge: Boydell, 2008.

McNally, Richard J., *Remembering Trauma*, Cambridge, MA: Harvard University Press, 2005.

Magot, Céline, "Elizabeth Bowen's London in *The Heat of the Day*: An Impression of the City in the Territory of War", *Literary London* III/1 (March 2005), <http://www.literarylondon.org/london journal/march2005/Magot.html>.

Malcolm, Cheryl Alexander, and David Malcolm, eds, *A Companion to the British and Irish Short Story*, Chichester: Wiley-Blackwell, 2008.

Mann, Chris, "Family Fables", in Chamberlain and Thompson, eds, *Narrative and Genre*, 81-98.

Mansergh, Martin, "Elizabeth Bowen and the Anglo-Irish Tradition", in Walshe, ed., *Elizabeth Bowen Remembered*, 40-50.

Marković, Vida E., *The Changing Face: Disintegration of Personality in the Twentieth-Century British Novel, 1900-1950*, Carbondale: Southern Illinois University Press, 1970.

Marrs, Suzanne, "Place and the Displaced in Eudora Welty's *The Bride of the Innisfallen*", *Mississippi Quarterly*, L/4 (Fall 1997), 647-68.

Martin, Augustine, "Literature and Society, 1938-51", in *Ireland in the War Years and After, 1939-51*, eds Kevin B. Nowlan and T. Desmond Williams, Dublin: Gill and Macmillan, 1969, 167-84.

Maslen, Elizabeth, "Women Writers in World War II", *Literature Compass*, III/3 (May 2006), 625-35.

—, *Political and Social Issues in British Women's Fiction, 1928-1968*, Houndmills: Palgrave, 2001.

Masschelein, Anneleen, "The Concept as Ghost: Conceptualization of the Uncanny in Late-Twentieth-Century Theory", *Mosaic*, IIIV/1 (March 2002), 53-68.

Mattison, Alice, "Jane Austen with Cigarettes", *Southwest Review*, LXXXIX/2-3 (2004), 282-92.

Mayrer, Rachel, "Gothic Memory and Forgetfulness in Elizabeth Bowen's *A World of Love* and 'The Demon Lover'", *Irish Studies Review*, XVI/1 (February 2008), 33-40.

Medoff, Jeslyn, "'There Is No Elsewhere': Elizabeth Bowen's Perceptions of War", *Modern Fiction Studies*, XXX/1 (Spring 1984), 73-81.

Mengham, Rod, "British Fiction of the War", in MacKay, ed., *The Cambridge Companion to the Literature of World War II*, 26-42.

Mengham, Rod, and N.H. Reeve, eds, *The Fiction of the 1940s: Stories of Survival*, Houndmills: Palgrave, 2001.

Mepham, John, "Varieties of Modernism, Varieties of Incomprehension: Patrick Hamilton and Elizabeth Bowen", in MacKay and Stonebridge, eds, *British Fiction after Modernism*, 59-76.

Micale, Mark S., and Paul Lerner, eds, *Traumatic Pasts: History, Psychiatry, and Trauma in the Modern Age, 1870-1930*, Cambridge: Cambridge University Press, 2001.

Middleton, Peter, and Tim Woods, *Literatures of Memory: History, Time and Space in Postwar Writing*, Manchester: Manchester University Press, 2000.

Miller, Brook, "The Impersonal Personal: Value, Voice, and Agency in Elizabeth Bowen's Literary and Social Criticism", *Modern Fiction Studies*, LIII/2 (Summer 2007), 351-69.

Miller, Brook, with Luke Elward, Tessa Hempel, and Philip Kollar, "Narrative, Meaning and Agency in *The Heat of the Day*", in Osborn, ed., *New Critical Perspectives*, 132-48.

Miller, Jane, "Re-Reading Elizabeth Bowen", *Raritan*, XX/1 (Summer 2000), 17-32.

Miller, J. Hillis, "Derrida's *Destinerrance*", *MLN*, CXXI/4 (September 2006), 893-910.

—, "Derrida's Remains", *Mosaic*, XXXIX/3 (September 2006), 197-211.

—, "Derrida's Topographies", *South Atlantic Review*, LIX/1 (January 1994), 1-25.

—, "Lying Against Death: Out of the Loop", in Jacobs and Sussman, eds, *Acts of Narrative*, 15-30.

—, *Ariadne's Thread: Story Lines*, New Haven, CT: Yale University Press, 1992.

—, *The Ethics of Reading: Kant, De Man, Eliot, Trollope, James, and Benjamin*, New York: Columbia University Press, 1987.
—, *Reading Narrative*, Norman: University of Oklahoma Press, 1998.
Miller, Kristine A., "'Even a Shelter's Not Safe': The Blitz on Homes in Elizabeth Bowen's Wartime Writing", *Twentieth Century Literature*, XLV/2 (Summer 1999), 138-58.
Miller, Nancy K., and Jason Daniel Tougaw, eds, *Extremities: Trauma, Testimony, and Community*, Chicago: University of Illinois Press, 2002.
Mitchell, Edward, "Themes in Elizabeth Bowen's Short Stories", in Bloom, ed., *Elizabeth Bowen*, 41-50.
Mitchell, Juliet, ed., *The Selected Melanie Klein*, Harmondsworth: Penguin, 1986.
Moi, Toril, *Sexual/Textual Politics: Feminist Literary Theory*, London: Methuen, 1985.
Montefiore, Janet, *Men and Women Writers of the 1930s: The Dangerous Flood of History*, London: Routledge, 1996.
Moody, T.W., "Review of *Bowen's Court*", *English Historical Review*, LX/237 (1945), 264-65.
Mooney, Sinéad, "Bowen and the Modern Ghost", in Walshe, ed., *Elizabeth Bowen*, 77-94.
—, "Unstable Compounds: Bowen's Beckettian Affinities", *Modern Fiction Studies*, LIII/2 (Summer 2007), 238-56.
Morrow, Ann, *Picnic in a Foreign Land: The Eccentric Lives of the Anglo-Irish*, London: Grafton, 1989.
Motte, Warren, "The Work of Mourning", *Yale French Studies*, CV (2004), 56-71.
Moynahan, Julian, *Anglo-Irish: The Literary Imagination in a Hyphenated Culture*, Princeton, NJ: Princeton University Press, 1995.
Muldoon, Paul, *To Ireland, I*, Oxford: Oxford University Press, 2000.
Muller, John P., and William J. Richardson, eds, *The Purloined Poe: Lacan, Derrida and Psychoanalytic Reading*, Baltimore, MD: Johns Hopkins University Press, 1988.
Munton, Alan, *English Fiction of the Second World War*, London: Faber and Faber, 1989.

Murphy, Sara, "Mourning and Metonymy: Bearing Witness Between Women and Generations", *Hypatia*, XIX/4 (Autumn 2004), 144-68.

Naas, Michael, "History's Remains: Of Memory, Mourning, and the Event", *Research in Phenomenology*, XXXIII/1 (January 2003), 75-96.

Naremore, James, *More Than Night: Film Noir in Its Contexts*, Berkeley: University of California Press, 1998.

Nicol, Bran, ed., *Postmodernism and the Contemporary Novel: A Reader*, Edinburgh: Edinburgh University Press, 2002.

Nicolas, Dominique, "*The Last September* by Elizabeth Bowen, or a Chronicle of a Foreshadowed Death", in *Back to the Present, Forward to the Past: Irish Writing and History since 1798*, eds Patricia A. Lynch, Joachim Fischer and Brian Coates, Amsterdam: Rodopi, 2006, 297-308.

Nora, Pierre, "Between Memory and History: *Les Lieux De Mémoire*", *Representations*, XXVI (Spring 1989), 7-24.

O'Faolain, Sean, *The Short Story*, London: Collins, 1948.

Oliver, Kelly, ed., *Ethics, Politics, and Difference in Julia Kristeva's Writing*, New York: Routledge, 1993.

Oppenheim, Janet, *The Other World: Spiritualism and Psychical Research in England, 1850-1914*, Cambridge: Cambridge University Press, 1985.

Osborn, Susan, "Elizabeth Bowen: New Directions for Critical Thinking", *Modern Fiction Studies*, LIII/2 (Summer 2007), 225-37.

—, "'How to Measure This Unaccountable Darkness Between the Trees': The Strange Relation of Style and Meaning in *The Last September*", in Osborn, ed., *New Critical Perspectives*, 34-60.

—, "Reconsidering Elizabeth Bowen", *Modern Fiction Studies*, LII/1 (Spring 2006), 187-98.

—, ed., *Elizabeth Bowen: New Critical Perspectives*, Togher: Cork UP, 2009.

O'Toole, Bridget, "Three Writers of the Big House: Elizabeth Bowen, Molly Keane and Jennifer Johnston", in *Across a Roaring Hill: The Protestant Imagination in Modern Ireland*, eds Gerald Dawe and Edna Longley, Belfast: Blackstaff, 1985, 124-38.

O'Toole, Tina, "Angels and Monsters: Embodiment and Desire in *Eva Trout*", in Walshe, ed., *Elizabeth Bowen*, 162-78.

Parkins, Wendy, "Moving Dangerously: Mobility and the Modern Woman", *Tulsa Studies in Women's Literature*, XX/1 (Spring 2001), 77-92.

Parsons, Deborah L., "Souls Astray: Elizabeth Bowen's Landscape of War", *Women: A Cultural Review*, VIII/1 (1997), 24-32.

—, *Streetwalking the Metropolis: Women, the City, and Modernity*, Oxford: Oxford University Press, 2000.

Peach, Linden, *The Contemporary Irish Novel: Critical Readings*, Houndmills: Palgrave Macmillan, 2004.

Peare, Oliver, with Molly Keane, "A Kinsale Perspective", in Walshe, ed., *Elizabeth Bowen Remembered*, 51-53.

Perce, Ann W., *Those Uneasy Currents: Elements of Menace and Terror in Selected Fiction of Elizabeth Bowen*, Boca Raton, FL: Universal, 2006.

Phillips, Lawrence, *London Narratives: Post-War Fiction and the City*, London: Continuum, 2006.

Piette, Adam, *Imagination at War: British Fiction and Poetry, 1939-45*, London: Papermac, 1995.

Plain, Gill, "From War-Time to Women's Time: Coping with Conflict in Women's Fiction of the 1940s", *Time & Society*, III/3 (October 1994), 341-64.

—, "Women Writers and the War", in MacKay, ed., *The Cambridge Companion to the Literature of World War II*, 165-78.

—, *Women's Fiction of the Second World War: Gender, Power and Resistance*, Edinburgh: Edinburgh University Press, 1996.

Poe, Edgar Allan, *Selected Tales* (1833-49), ed. David van Leer, Oxford: Oxford University Press, 1998.

Pong, Beryl, "Space and Time in the Bombed City: Graham Greene's *The Ministry of Fear* and Elizabeth Bowen's *The Heat of the Day*", *Literary London*, VII/1 (March 2009) <http://www.literary london.org/london-journal/pong.html>.

Priestman, Martin, *Crime Fiction from Poe to the Present*, Plymouth: Northcote House, 1998.

Proctor, Tammy M., *Female Intelligence: Women and Espionage in the First World War*, New York: New York University Press, 2003.

Punter, David, ed., *A Companion to the Gothic*, Oxford: Blackwell, 2001.

Pyle, Hilary, "A Portrait of Elizabeth Bowen by Patrick Hennessy", in Walshe, ed., *Elizabeth Bowen Remembered*, 54-59.

Quinn, Patrick J., ed., *Recharting the Thirties*, Selinsgrove, PA: Susquehanna University Press, 1996.

Quinn, Patrick J., and Steven Trout, eds, *The Literature of the Great War Reconsidered: Beyond Modern Memory*, Houndmills: Palgrave, 2001.

Radford, Jean, "Face to Face with the Other: Levinas and Elizabeth Bowen's *The House in Paris*", in *Modernity, Modernism, Postmodernism*, ed. Manuel Barbeito, Santiago de Compostela: Universidade Servicio de Publicacións e Intercambio Cientiífico, 2000, 93-106.

—, "Late Modernism and the Politics of History", in Joannou, ed., *Women Writers of the 1930s*, 33-45

Raitt, Suzanne, and Trudi Tate, eds, *Women's Fiction and the Great War*, Oxford: Oxford University Press, 1997.

Ramazani, Jahan, *Poetry of Mourning: The Modern Elegy from Hardy to Heaney*, Chicago: University of Chicago Press, 1994.

Rand, Nicholas T., and Maria Torok, "The Secret of Psychoanalysis: History Reads Theory", *Critical Inquiry*, XIII/2 (Winter 1987), 278-86.

Randall, Phyllis R., "Pinter and Bowen: *The Heat of the Day*", in *Pinter at Sixty*, eds Katherine H. Burkman and John L. Kundert-Gibbs, Bloomington: Indiana University Press, 1993, 173-82.

Rashkin, Esther, *Family Secrets and the Psychoanalysis of Narrative*, Princeton, NJ: Princeton University Press, 1992.

Rau, Petra, "The Common Frontier: Fictions of Alterity in Elizabeth Bowen's *The Heat of the Day* and Graham Greene's *The Ministry of Fear*", *Literature and History*, XIV/1 (Spring 2005), 31-55.

Rauchbauer, Otto, ed., *Ancestral Voices: The Big House in Anglo-Irish Literature*, Hildesheim: Georg Olms Verlag, 1992.

Rawlinson, Mark, *British Writing of the Second World War*, Oxford: Clarendon, 2000.

Raymond, Claire, *The Posthumous Voice in Women's Writing from Mary Shelley to Sylvia Plath*, Aldershot: Ashgate, 2006.

Reynolds, Lorna, "*The Last September* – Elizabeth Bowen's Paradise Lost", in Rauchbauer, ed., *Ancestral Voices*, 149-58.

Rich, Adrienne, *Of Woman Born: Motherhood as Experience and Institution*, London: Virago, 1977.

Rickels, Laurence A., *Aberrations of Mourning: Writing on German Crypts*, Detroit, MI: Wayne State University Press, 1988.

Ricoeur, Paul, *Memory, History, Forgetting*, trans. Kathleen Blamey and David Pellauer, Chicago: University of Chicago Press, 2004.

—, *The Rule of Metaphor: Multi-Disciplinary Studies of the Creation of Meaning in Language*, trans. Robert Czerny, Kathleen McLaughlin and John Costello, London: Routledge and Kegan Paul, 1978.

—, *Time and Narrative*, trans. Kathleen McLaughlin and David Pellauer, Vol. I, Chicago: University of Chicago Press, 1984.

—, *Time and Narrative*, trans. Kathleen McLaughlin and David Pellauer, Vol. II, Chicago: University of Chicago Press, 1985.

Robbins, Michael, "Another Look at Dreaming: Disentangling Freud's Primary and Secondary Process Theories", *JAPA*, LII/2 (June 2004), 355-84.

Robson, Kathryn, *Writing Wounds: The Inscription of Trauma in post-1968 French Women's Life-Writing*, Amsterdam: Rodopi, 2004.

Rose, Jacqueline, "Bizarre Objects: Mary Butts and Elizabeth Bowen", *Critical Quarterly*, XLII/1 (April 2000), 75-85.

—, *On Not Being Able to Sleep: Psychoanalysis and the Modern World*, London: Chatto and Windus, 2003.

—, *Why War? Psychoanalysis, Politics, and the Return to Melanie Klein*, Oxford: Blackwell, 1993.

Rothberg, Michael, *Traumatic Realism: The Demands of Holocaust Representation*, Minneapolis: University of Minnesota Press, 2000.

Royle, Nicholas, "Portmanteau", *New Literary History*, XXXVII/1 (Winter 2006), 237-47.

—, "The 'Telepathy Effect': Notes Toward a Reconsideration of Narrative Fiction", in Jacobs and Sussman, eds, *Acts of Narrative*, 93-109.

—, *After Derrida*, Manchester: Manchester University Press, 1995.

—, *Jacques Derrida*, London: Routledge, 2003.

—, *Telepathy and Literature: Essays on the Reading Mind*, Oxford: Basil Blackwell, 1991.

—, *The Uncanny*, Manchester: Manchester University Press, 2003.

Ruddick, Sara, "Maternal Thinking", *Feminist Studies*, VI/2 (Summer 1980), 342-67.

Rumbarger, Lee, "Housekeeping: Women Modernists' Writing on War and Home", *Women's Studies*, XXXV/1 (January-February 2006), 1-15.

Sacks, Peter, *The English Elegy: Studies in Genre from Spenser to Yeats*, Baltimore, MD: Johns Hopkins University Press, 1985.

Sage, Victor, "Irish Gothic: C.R. Maturin and J.S. Le Fanu", in Punter, ed., *A Companion to the Gothic*, 81-93.

Santner, Eric L., *Stranded Objects: Mourning, Memory, and Film in Postwar Germany*, Ithaca, NY: Cornell University Press, 1990.

Sayers, Janet, *Sexual Contradictions: Psychology, Psychoanalysis, and Feminism*, London: Tavistock, 1986.

Scanlan, Margaret, "The Recuperation of History in British and Irish Fiction", in Shaffer, ed., *A Companion to the British and Irish Novel*, 144-59.

—, "Rumours of War: Elizabeth Bowen's *The Last September* and J.G. Farrell's *Troubles*", *Eire-Ireland*, XX/2 (Summer 1985), 70-89.

Sceats, Sarah, "Souls Astray: Belonging and the Idea of Home: Elizabeth Bowen's *The Heat of the Day*, Betty Miller's *On the Side of the Angels*, and *Death of the Nightingale*, and Muriel Spark's *Memento Mori*", in Dowson, ed., *Women's Writing*, 85-97.

Sceats, Sarah, and Gail Cunningham, eds, *Image and Power: Women in Fiction in the Twentieth Century*, London: Longman, 1996.

Schafer, Roy, "Narration in the Psychoanalytic Dialogue", *Critical Quarterly*, VII/1 (Autumn 1980), 29-53.

Schama, Simon, *Landscape and Memory* (1995), London: Harper Perennial, 2004.

Schneidau, Herbert N., *Waking Giants: The Presence of the Past in Modernism*, Oxford: Oxford University Press, 1991.

Schneider, Karen, *Loving Arms: British Women Writing the Second World War*, Lexington: University Press of Kentucky, 1997.

Schor, Esther, *Bearing the Dead: The British Culture of Mourning from the Enlightenment to Victoria*, Princeton, NJ: Princeton University Press, 1994.

Schwab, Gabriele, "Writing Against Memory and Forgetting",

Literature and Medicine, XXV/1 (Spring 2006), 95-121.

Schwartz, Louis-Georges, "Cinema and the ~~Meaning~~ of 'Life'", *Discourse*, XXVIII/2-3 (Spring-Fall 2006), 7-27.

Sellery, J. Nan, and William O. Harris, *Elizabeth Bowen: A Bibliography*, Austin: University of Texas Press, 1981.

Seward, Barbara, "Elizabeth Bowen's World of Impoverished Love", *College English*, XVIII/1 (October 1956), 30-37.

Shaffer, Brian W., ed., *A Companion to the British and Irish Novel, 1945-2000*, Malden, MA: Blackwell, 2005.

Shaw, Valerie, *The Short Story: A Critical Introduction*, London: Longman, 1983.

Showalter, Elaine, *A Literature of Their Own: British Women Novelists from Bronte to Lessing*, rev. edn, London: Virago, 1982.

Shumaker, Jeanette, "Bruised Boys and 'Fallen' Women: The Need for Rescue in Short Stories by Elizabeth Bowen", *South Carolina Review*, XXXII/1 (Fall 1999), 88-98.

Sinfield, Alan, *Literature, Politics and Culture in Postwar Britain*, 2nd edn, London: Continuum, 2004.

Sokolsky, Anita, "The Melancholy Persuasion", in Ellmann, ed., *Psychoanalytic Literary Criticism*, 128-42.

Spooner, Catherine, and Emma McEvoy, eds, *The Routledge Companion to Gothic*, Abingdon: Routledge, 2007.

Stevens, Julie Anne, "Bowen: The Critical Response", in Walshe, ed., *Elizabeth Bowen*, 179-92.

Stewart, Pamela J., and Andrew Strathern, eds, *Landscape, Memory and History: Anthropological Perspectives*, London: Pluto, 2003.

Stewart, Victoria, "'That Eternal "Now"': Memory and Subjectivity in Elizabeth Bowen's *Seven Winters*", *Modern Fiction Studies*, LIII/2 (Summer 2007), 334-50.

—, "Violence and Representation in Elizabeth Bowen's Interwar Short Stories", *English*, LVIII/221 (Summer 2009), 139-59.

—, *Narratives of Memory: British Writing of the 1940s*, Houndmills: Palgrave Macmillan, 2006.

—, *Women's Autobiography: War and Trauma*, Houndmills: Palgrave Macmillan, 2003.

Stonebridge, Lyndsey, "Anxiety at a Time of Crisis", *History Workshop Journal*, XLV (Spring 1998), 171-82.

—, "Bombs and Roses: The Writing of Anxiety in Henry Green's 'Caught'", *Diacritics*, XXVIII/4 (Winter 1998), 25-43.

—, "Theories of Trauma", in MacKay, *The Cambridge Companion to the Literature of World War II*, 194-206.

—, *The Writing of Anxiety: Imagining Wartime in Mid-Century British Culture*, Houndmills: Palgrave Macmillan, 2007.

Sturrock, June, "Mumbo-Jumbo: The Haunted World of *The Little Girls*", in Osborn, ed., *New Critical Perspectives*, 83-95.

Suleiman, Susan Rubin, *Crises of Memory and the Second World War*, Cambridge, MA: Harvard University Press, 2006.

Sullivan, Walter, "A Sense of Place: Elizabeth Bowen and the Landscape of the Heart", *Sewanee Review*, LXXXIV/1 (1976), 142-49.

Summers-Bremner, Eluned, "Dead Letters and Living Things: Historical Ethics in *The House in Paris* and *The Death of the Heart*", in Osborn, ed., *New Critical Perspectives*, 61-82.

—, "Heart(h) and Home: Elizabeth Bowen's Irishness", *Études Irlandaises*, XXIX/2 (Summer 2004), 135-50.

—, "Monumental City: Elizabeth Bowen and the Modern Unhomely", in *Modernism and Mourning*, ed. Patricia Rae, Harrisburg, PA: Bucknell University Press, 2006, 260-69.

Sword, Helen, *Ghostwriting Modernism*, Ithaca, NY: Cornell University Press, 2002.

Tatum, James, *The Mourner's Song: War and Remembrance from the Iliad to Vietnam*, Chicago: University of Chicago Press, 2003.

Taxidou, Olga, *Tragedy, Modernity and Mourning*, Edinburgh: Edinburgh University Press, 2004.

Thompson, Terry W., "'The Demon Lover': Elizabeth Bowen's 'Unashamed Retelling' of 'The Jolly Corner'", *South Carolina Review*, XXXIX/1 (September 2006), 57-65.

Thurschwell, Adam, "Writing and Terror: Don DeLillo on the Task of Literature after 9/11", *Law and Literature*, XIX/2 (Summer 2007), 277-302.

Thurschwell, Pamela, "Ferenczi's Dangerous Proximities: Telepathy, Psychosis, and the Real Event", *Differences*, XI/1 (Spring 1999), 150-78.

Tillinghast, Richard, "Elizabeth Bowen: The House, the Hotel, and the Child", *New Criterion*, XIII/4 (December 1994), 24-33.

Toremans, Tom, “Trauma: Theory – Reading (and) Literary Theory in the Wake of Trauma”, *European Journal of English Studies*, VII/3 (2003), 333-51.

Towheed, Shafquat, “Territory, Space, Modernity: Elizabeth Bowen’s *The Demon Lover and Other Stories* and Wartime London”, in Osborn, ed., *New Critical Perspectives*, 113-31.

Tracy, Robert, “Undead, Unburied: Anglo-Ireland and the Predatory Past”, *LIT*, X/1 (July 1999), 13-33.

Trezise, Thomas, “Between History and Psychoanalysis: A Case Study in the Reception of Holocaust Survivor Testimony”, *History and Memory*, XX/1 (Spring-Summer 2008), 7-47.

Trigg, Dylan, “The Place of Trauma: Memory, Hauntings, and the Temporality of Ruins”, *Memory Studies*, II/1 (January 2009), 87-101.

—, *The Aesthetics of Decay: Nothingness, Nostalgia, and the Absence of Reason*, New York: Peter Lang, 2006.

Trotter, David, *Cooking with Mud: The Idea of Mess in Nineteenth-Century Art and Fiction*, Oxford: Oxford University Press, 2000.

Turim, Maureen, *Flashback in Film: Memory and History*, New York: Routledge, 1989.

Tylee, Claire M., *The Great War and Women’s Consciousness: Images of Militarism and Womanhood in Women’s Writings, 1914-64*, Houndmills: Macmillan, 1990.

Van Duyn, Mona, “Pattern and Pilgrimage: A Reading of *The Death of the Heart*”, in Bloom, ed., *Elizabeth Bowen*, 13-25 .

Vernadakis, Emmanuel, “Christening Pagans: Onomastics and Plot in Elizabeth Bowen’s ‘Daffodils’, ‘Her Table Spread’ and ‘Look At All Those Roses’”, *Journal of the Short Story in English*, XXXIV (Spring 2000), 2-14.

Vickroy, Laurie, *Trauma and Survival in Contemporary Fiction*, Charlottesville: University of Virginia Press, 2002.

Vidler, Anthony, *The Architectural Uncanny: Essays in the Modern Unhomely*, Cambridge, MA: MIT Press, 1992.

Wagner, Geoffrey, “Elizabeth Bowen and the Artificial Novel”, *Essays in Criticism*, XIII/2 (April 1963), 155-63.

Walker, Janet, *Trauma Cinema: Documenting Incest and the Holocaust*, Berkeley: University of California Press, 2005.

Wallace, Diana, "Uncanny Stories: The Ghost Story as Female Gothic", *Gothic Studies*, VI/1 (May 2004), 57-69.

Walsh, Keri, "Elizabeth Bowen, Surrealist", *Eire-Ireland*, XLII/3-4 (Fall-Winter 2007), 126-47.

Walshe, Eibhear, "'A Lout's Game': Espionage, Irishness, and Sexuality in *The Untouchable*", *Irish University Review* XXXVI/1 (Spring-Summer 2006), 102-16.

—, "Several Landscapes: Bowen and the Terrain of North Cork", *Estudios Irlandeses*, 0 (2005), 141-47.

—, "A Sort of Lunatic Giant", in Walshe, ed., *Elizabeth Bowen*, 150-61.

—, "A Time for Hard Writers", in Walshe, ed., *Elizabeth Bowen*, 95-109.

—, ed., *Elizabeth Bowen Remembered: The Farahy Addresses*, Dublin: Four Courts, 1998.

—, ed., *Elizabeth Bowen*, Dublin: Irish Academic Press, 2009.

—, ed., *Sex, Nation and Dissent in Irish Writing*, Cork: Cork University Press, 1997.

Warner, Alan, *A Guide to Anglo-Irish Literature*, Dublin: Gill and Macmillan, 1981.

Warren, Victoria, "'Experience Means Nothing Till It Repeats Itself': Elizabeth Bowen's *The Death of the Heart* and Jane Austen's *Emma*", *Modern Language Studies*, XXIX/1 (Spring 1999), 131-54.

Watson, Barbara Bellow, "Variations on an Enigma: Elizabeth Bowen's War Novel", in Bloom, ed., *Elizabeth Bowen*, 81-101.

Weekes, Ann Owens, *Irish Women Writers: An Uncharted Tradition*, Lexington, KY: University Press of Kentucky, 1990.

Wells-Lassagne, Shannon, "He Believed in Empire: Colonial Concerns in Elizabeth Bowen's *The Last September*", *Irish Studies Review*, XV/4 (2007), 451-63.

—, "'*She*-ward Bound': Elizabeth Bowen as a Sensationalist Writer", in Osborn, ed., *New Critical Perspectives*, 96-112.

Wessels, Andries, "Elizabeth Bowen's *A World of Love*: A 'Cultural Analysis' of the Anglo-Irish Ascendancy in the Twentieth Century", *Canadian Journal of Irish Studies*, XXI/1 (July 1995), 88-95.

Whitehead, Anne, *Memory*, Oxford: Routledge, 2009.

—, *Trauma Fiction*, Edinburgh: Edinburgh University Press, 2004.

Whitworth, Michael H., *Einstein's Wake: Relativity, Metaphor, and Modernist Literature*, Oxford: Oxford University Press, 2001.

Wightman, Beth, "Geopolitics and the Sight of the Nation: Elizabeth Bowen's *The Last September*", *LIT*, XVIII/1 (2007), 37-64.

Williams, Julia McElhattan, "'Fiction with the Texture of History': Elizabeth Bowen's *The Last September*", *Modern Fiction Studies*, XLI/2 (Summer 1995), 219-42.

Wills, Clair, "The Aesthetics of Irish Neutrality During the Second World War", *Boundary 2*, XXXI/1 (Spring 2004), 119-45.

—, "'Half Different': The Vanishing Irish in *A World of Love*", in Walshe, ed., *Elizabeth Bowen*, 133-49.

—, *That Neutral Island: A Cultural History of Ireland During the Second World War*, London: Faber and Faber, 2007.

Winter, Jay, *Sites of Memory, Sites of Mourning: The Great War in European Cultural History*, Cambridge: Cambridge University Press, 1995.

Winter, Jay, and Emmanuel Sivan, eds, *War and Remembrance in the Twentieth Century*, Cambridge: Cambridge University Press, 1999.

Wolff, Ellen M., *"An Anarchy in the Mind and in the Heart": Narrating Anglo-Ireland*, Harrisburg, PA: Bucknell University Press, 2006.

Wolfreys, Julian, *Readings: Acts of Close Reading in Literary Theory*, Edinburgh: Edinburgh University Press, 2000.

Wood, Nancy, *Vectors of Memory: Legacies of Trauma in Postwar Europe*, Oxford: Berg, 1999.

Wright, Elizabeth, *Psychoanalytic Criticism: A Reappraisal*, 2nd edn, Cambridge: Polity, 1998.

Wyatt-Brown, Anne M., "The Liberation of Mourning in Elizabeth Bowen's *The Little Girls* and *Eva Trout*", in *Aging and Gender in Literature: Studies in Creativity*, eds Anne M. Wyatt-Brown and Janice Rossen, Charlottesville: University of Virginia Press, 1993, 164-86.

York, R.A., *The Rules of Time: Time and Rhythm in the Twentieth-Century Novel*, Cranbury, NJ: Associated University Presses, 1999.

Zelizer, Barbie, *Remembering to Forget: Holocaust Memory Through the Camera's Eye*, Chicago: University of Chicago Press, 1998.

INDEX

www.ingramcontent.com/pod-product-compliance
Lightning Source LLC
Chambersburg PA
CBHW031323230926
51848CB00001B/63